Overcoming
Endometrial Cancer

An In-Depth Guide to Understanding Its Causes, Symptoms, Advanced Treatments, and Effective Prevention Strategies for Recovery.

(Things You Must Know)

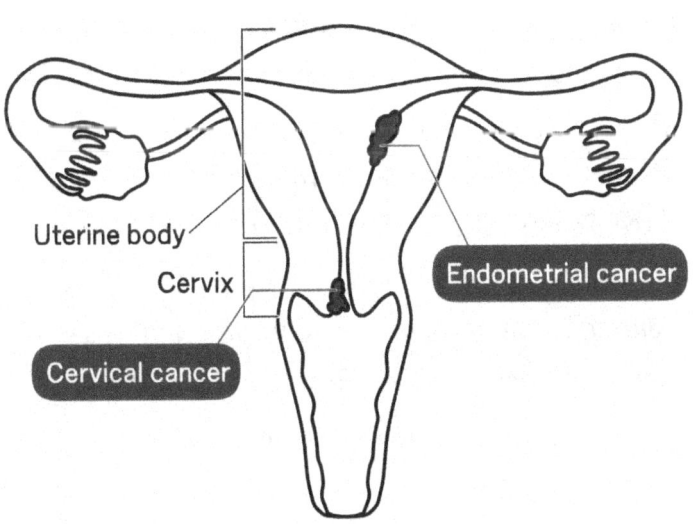

Isabella White

Disclaimer: The information in this book is based on the author's research and experiences. It is not intended to replace professional medical advice. Always consult a physician for any health issues before modifying diet, supplements, or exercise regimens. The author and publisher have no liability or responsibility for any loss or damage related to the information contained in this book. Any reliance on this information is solely at the reader's risk.

Table of Contents

Introduction

Endometrial cancer, also known as uterine cancer, is a condition that affects the uterus and requires prompt medical attention. As the most common gynecological cancer in the United States, an estimated 65,950 women were diagnosed with endometrial cancer in 2023 alone.

Endometrial cancer can cause symptoms such as abnormal vaginal bleeding, pelvic pain, and difficulty urinating. If detected early, endometrial cancer can be treated with surgery, radiation, chemotherapy, hormone therapy, or a combination of these options. However, some women may face challenges such as recurrence, side effects, or emotional distress after treatment.

This book provides an in-depth guide to understanding the causes, symptoms, advanced treatments, and effective prevention strategies for endometrial cancer. Whether you are a patient, a caregiver, a doctor, or a curious reader, this book will equip you with the knowledge and tools you need to cope with and overcome this disease. You will learn about:

- The risk factors and possible causes of endometrial cancer include genetics, hormones, obesity, diabetes, and inflammation.
- The signs and symptoms of endometrial cancer and how to recognize them early.
- The diagnostic tests and procedures for endometrial cancer, such as pelvic exams, biopsy, ultrasound, MRI, CT scans, and PET scans.
- The staging and grading systems for endometrial cancer and what they mean for your prognosis and treatment plan.
- The treatment options and guidelines for endometrial cancer include surgery, radiation, chemotherapy, hormone therapy, immunotherapy, and targeted therapy.

- The benefits and risks of each treatment option and how to prepare for them.
- The possible complications and side effects of treatment, such as infection, bleeding, lymphedema, infertility, menopause, sexual dysfunction, and neuropathy.
- The follow-up care and surveillance for endometrial cancer and how to prevent recurrence or metastasis.
- The prevention strategies and lifestyle changes for endometrial cancer include diet, exercise, weight management, stress reduction, and screening.
- The emotional and psychological aspects of endometrial cancer and how to cope with them.
- The support and resources available for endometrial cancer patients, caregivers, and survivors include online communities, support groups, counseling, and financial assistance.

This book will give you a comprehensive and holistic understanding of endometrial cancer and how to deal with it effectively. You will also find hope and inspiration from women who have faced and overcome this disease. This book is intended to complement, not replace, advice from healthcare providers, empowering informed decisions about health and well-being.

I hope this book will help you overcome endometrial cancer and that you will find it helpful and informative. Thank you for choosing this book, and I wish you all the best.

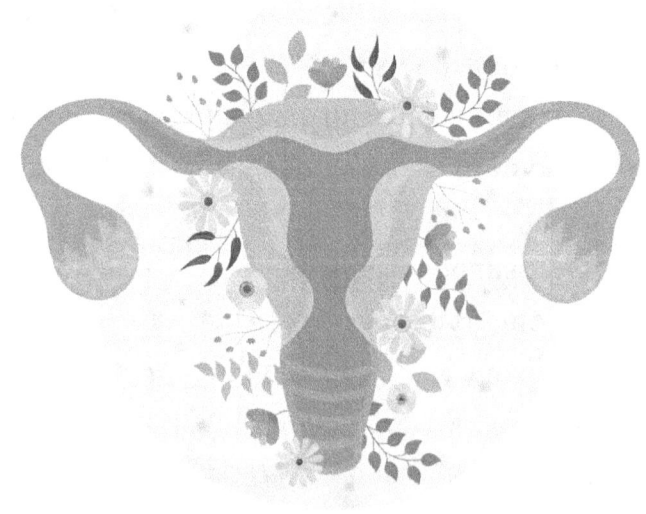

ENDOMETRIOSIS

Chapter 1

The Basics of Endometrial Cancer

What is Endometrial Cancer?

Endometrial cancer begins when healthy cells in the lining of the uterus, known as the endometrium, start to grow out of control. As these cancerous cells rapidly multiply, they can form a mass of tissue called a tumor in the uterus.

The most common type of endometrial cancer is adenocarcinoma. This begins in the glandular cells that make the uterine lining thick and nutritious in preparation for pregnancy. Suppose adenocarcinoma is not diagnosed and treated early. In that case, it can spread from the endometrium's surface into the uterus's deeper tissues. Cancer cells may reach the lymph nodes, bloodstream, or pelvic organs from there.

UTERINE FIBROIDS

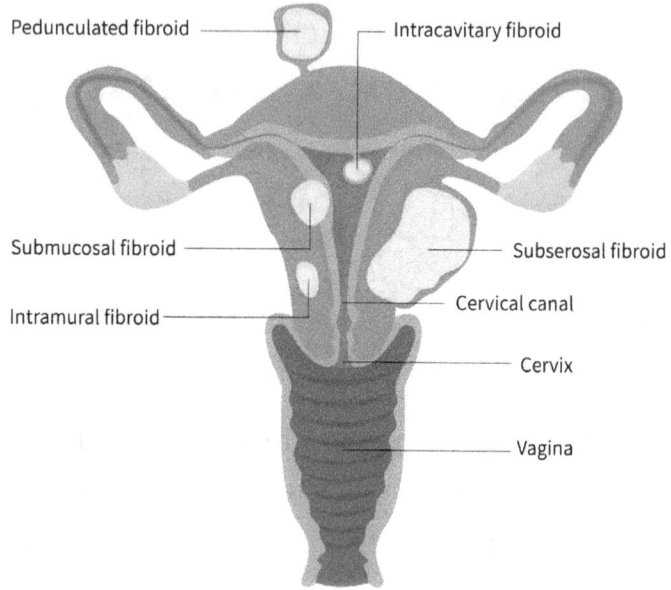

While endometrial cancer often stays confined to the uterus in its early stages, the risk of it spreading grows over time. That's why early detection and treatment provide the best chance for survival. Catching it before cancer cells have invaded deeper uterine layers or spread outside the uterus improves the prognosis significantly.

What makes a woman develop endometrial cancer? The hormones estrogen and progesterone drive the growth of the endometrium each month to build the uterine lining. When the balance of these hormones is disrupted, it can spur abnormal cell growth that may become cancerous over time.

Risk factors like starting menstruation early, entering menopause late, having no children, obesity, diabetes, breast cancer, and using estrogen therapy without progesterone can all impact hormone levels and raise endometrial cancer risks. Women with Lynch syndrome, also known as hereditary nonpolyposis colorectal cancer (HNPCC), also have an increased risk.

While endometrial cancer often has no obvious early symptoms, signs like abnormal vaginal bleeding, pelvic pain or pressure, and pain during intercourse may be present as the cancer progresses. That's why it's critical that women, especially post-menopausal women experiencing vaginal bleeding, see a doctor promptly for evaluation.

Detecting endometrial cancer begins with a pelvic exam, Pap test, and transvaginal ultrasound. If abnormalities are found, a biopsy of the uterine lining will be done to analyze the cells and confirm a cancer diagnosis. Once diagnosed, staging tests help determine how advanced the cancer is so that an optimal treatment plan can be developed.

The Anatomy of the Endometrium

The endometrium is the inner lining of the uterus, the hollow, pear-shaped organ where a baby grows during pregnancy. The endometrium is made up of two layers: the basal layer and the functional layer.

The basal layer is the deeper layer that attaches to the muscular wall of the uterus, called the myometrium. The basal layer comprises a single layer of columnar epithelial cells and an underlying layer of connective tissue called the stroma. The stroma contains blood vessels, lymphatic vessels, nerves, and immune cells. The basal layer serves as the source of regeneration for the functional layer and remains relatively constant throughout the menstrual cycle.

The functional layer is the superficial layer that faces the uterine cavity. The functional layer is also composed of columnar epithelial cells and stroma but has additional structures called uterine glands. The uterine glands are tubular glands that secrete mucus and other substances to nourish the embryo and the placenta. The functional layer undergoes cyclic changes in response to the hormones estrogen and progesterone produced by the ovaries. The functional layer is the part of the endometrium where fertilized egg implantation occurs and the placenta develops.

The functional layer can be divided into two sublayers: the stratum compactum and the spongiosum. The stratum compactum is the thin, outermost sublayer adjacent to the epithelium. It contains densely packed stromal cells and a few glands. The stratum spongiosum is the thick, innermost sublayer adjacent to the basal layer. It contains loosely arranged stromal cells and numerous glands.

The thickness and structure of the functional layer vary throughout the menstrual cycle, which can be divided into four phases: the menstrual phase, the proliferative phase, the secretory phase, and the ischemic phase.

The menstrual phase lasts about 3 to 7 days and occurs when the functional layer is shed as menstrual blood. This happens when the levels of estrogen and progesterone drop due to the absence of pregnancy. The menstrual blood consists of blood, tissue, mucus, and bacteria. The basal layer remains intact and serves as the foundation for the next cycle.

The proliferative phase lasts about 9 to 10 days and occurs when the functional layer is rebuilt under the influence of estrogen. The estrogen is produced by the growing follicles in the ovaries, which are the structures that contain the eggs. The epithelial and stromal cells multiply, and the uterine glands elongate. The blood vessels also grow and branch. The endometrium becomes thicker and more vascularized. The proliferative phase ends with ovulation, which is the release of the egg from the ovary.

The secretory phase lasts about 14 days and occurs when the functional layer is prepared for implantation under the influence of progesterone.

Progesterone is produced by the corpus luteum, which is the structure that forms from the ruptured follicle after ovulation. The epithelial cells and the stromal cells become larger and more active. The uterine glands secrete glycogen and other substances to nourish the potential embryo. The blood vessels become more coiled and dilated. The endometrium reaches its maximum thickness and secretory activity. The secretory phase ends with the degeneration of the corpus luteum unless pregnancy occurs.

The ischemic phase lasts about 1 to 2 days and occurs when the functional layer is deprived of blood supply and oxygen. This happens when the levels of estrogen and progesterone drop due to the degeneration of the corpus luteum. The blood vessels constrict and rupture, causing bleeding and tissue death. The epithelial and stromal cells disintegrate and detach from the basal layer. The ischemic phase leads to the onset of the menstrual phase, and the cycle repeats.

The primary function of the endometrium is to provide a suitable environment for the implantation and development of the embryo. The endometrium also prevents the adhesion of the uterus's opposite walls and maintains the uterine cavity's patency. The endometrium is influenced by hormones, genetics, inflammation, and infection, affecting its structure and function.

How Common is Endometrial Cancer?

Endometrial cancer is the most common cancer of the female reproductive organs in the United States. According to the American Cancer Society, about 67,880 new cases of cancer of the uterus will be diagnosed in 2024, and about 13,250 women will die from it. These estimates include both endometrial cancers and uterine sarcomas, which are rare types of uterine cancer that start in the muscle or connective tissue of the uterus. Up to 10% of uterine cancers are sarcomas, so the actual numbers for endometrial cancer cases and deaths are slightly lower than these estimates.

Endometrial cancer affects mainly post-menopausal women, with the average age at diagnosis being 60. However, it can also occur in younger women, especially those who have certain risk factors or genetic conditions. Endometrial cancer is more common in Black women than in White women, and Black women are more likely to die from it.

The incidence and mortality rates of endometrial cancer have been increasing over the past decade by about 1% per year in White women and 2% to 3% per year in women of all other racial and ethnic groups. This may be due to several factors, such as the rising rates of obesity, diabetes, and estrogen exposure, which are known to increase the risk of endometrial cancer. Other factors, such as environmental exposures, lifestyle habits, and access to health care, may also play a role.

Endometrial cancer is usually curable if detected early, but it can also be life-threatening if it progresses or recurs. The survival rates for endometrial cancer depend on several factors, such as the stage, grade, type, and location of the cancer, as well as the age, health, and treatment of the patient.

The 5-year relative survival rate for all stages of endometrial cancer is about 81%, meaning that women with endometrial cancer are, on average, about 81% as likely as women without the cancer to live for at least five years after being diagnosed. However, the survival rates vary widely by stage, from 95% for localized cancers (confined to the uterus) to 17% for distant cancers (spread to other parts of the body).

There are more than 600,000 survivors of endometrial cancer in the US today. Survivors may face challenges such as recurrence, side effects, or emotional distress after treatment. They may also need regular follow-up care and surveillance to monitor their health and prevent complications. In the later chapters, we will discuss the treatment options and guidelines, the follow-up care and surveillance, and the coping strategies and resources for endometrial cancer patients, caregivers, and survivors.

Stages and Grades of Endometrial Cancer

Endometrial cancer is a heterogeneous disease, meaning it can have different characteristics and behaviors depending on the type, stage, and grade of the cancer. These factors can help doctors determine each patient's prognosis and treatment options.

The type of endometrial cancer refers to the type of cell or tissue that the cancer originated from. The most common type of endometrial cancer is endometrioid adenocarcinoma, which accounts for about 80% of cases. This type of cancer arises from the glandular cells of the endometrium. Other types of endometrial cancer include:

- **Uterine serous carcinoma:** This type of cancer accounts for about 10% of cases. It arises from the surface cells of the endometrium and tends to be more aggressive and resistant to treatment than endometrioid adenocarcinoma.
- **Clear cell carcinoma:** This type of cancer accounts for about 4% of cases. It arises from the surface cells of the endometrium and has a clear appearance under the microscope. It is also more aggressive and resistant to treatment than endometrioid adenocarcinoma.
- **Carcinosarcoma:** This type of cancer accounts for about 4% of cases. It has features of both endometrial cancer and sarcoma, a

cancer of the connective tissue. It is also very aggressive and resistant to treatment.

- **Other rare types:** These include squamous cell carcinoma, small cell carcinoma, transitional cell carcinoma, and mixed cell carcinoma.

The stage of endometrial cancer describes how far the cancer has spread within the uterus or beyond it. The staging system used for endometrial cancer is based on the TNM system, which stands for tumor, node, and metastasis. The tumor (T) category describes how deep the cancer has grown into the uterus or nearby structures. The node (N) category describes whether the cancer has spread to nearby lymph nodes. The metastasis (M) category describes whether the cancer has spread to distant organs or tissues. Based on these categories, endometrial cancer is divided into four stages, from I to IV. The lower the stage, the less the cancer has spread and the better the prognosis.

The table below summarizes the TNM categories and the corresponding stages for endometrial cancer:

T category	N category	M category	Stage
T1a: The cancer is limited to the endometrium or less than half of the myometrium	N0: No spread to nearby lymph nodes	M0: No spread to distant sites	Stage IA
T1b: The cancer has invaded more than half of the myometrium	N0	M0	Stage IB
T2: The cancer has spread to the cervix, but not beyond the uterus	N0	M0	Stage II
T3a: The cancer has spread to the outer layer of the uterus (serosa) or the fallopian tubes or ovaries	N0	M0	Stage IIIA
T3b: The cancer has spread to the vagina or the parametrium (the tissue around the uterus)	N0	M0	Stage IIIB
Any T	N1: The cancer has spread to the pelvic lymph nodes	M0	Stage IIIC1
Any T	N2: The cancer has spread to the para-aortic lymph nodes	M0	Stage IIIC2
T4: The cancer has spread to the bladder or the bowel	Any N	M0	Stage IVA
Any T	Any N	M1: The cancer has spread to distant sites, such	Stage IVB

		as the lungs, liver, or bones	

The grade of endometrial cancer describes how abnormal the cancer cells look under the microscope. The grade shows how fast the cancer cells are growing and dividing. The grading system used for endometrial cancer is based on the degree of differentiation, which is how much the cancer cells resemble normal endometrial cells.

Based on this, endometrial cancer is divided into three grades, from G1 to G3. The lower the grade, the more differentiated the cancer cells are and the better the prognosis. The table below summarizes the grading system for endometrial cancer:

Grade	Description
G1: Well differentiated.	The cancer cells look very similar to normal endometrial cells. They tend to grow slowly and have a low risk of spreading.
G2: Moderately differentiated.	The cancer cells look somewhat different from normal endometrial cells. They tend to grow faster and risk spreading more than G1 cancers.
G3: Poorly differentiated.	The cancer cells look very different from normal endometrial cells. They tend to grow rapidly and have a high risk of spreading.

Statistics and Prevalence

Statistics and prevalence are two ways of measuring how widespread a disease is. Statistics are numerical data that describe the frequency, distribution, and trends of a disease in a population. Prevalence is the proportion of people with the disease at a given time or over time. Here, You will see statistics and prevalence data for endometrial cancer globally and in the United States.

Global statistics and prevalence

According to the World Cancer Research Fund International, endometrial cancer is the sixth most common cancer in women worldwide and the 15th most common cancer overall. There were more than 417,000 new cases of endometrial cancer in 2020, accounting for about 2.8% of all new cancer cases. The global age-standardized incidence rate (ASR) of endometrial cancer was 8.7 per 100,000 women in 2020. The ASR is a summary measure of the rate of disease that adjusts for the differences in age structure among populations.

The global distribution of endometrial cancer is uneven, with some regions having higher or lower rates than others. The highest ASRs of endometrial cancer in 2020 were found in Eastern Europe (18.9 per 100,000 women), Northern America (16.5 per 100,000 women), and Western Europe (15.4 per 100,000 women). The lowest ASRs of endometrial cancer in 2020 were found in Middle Africa (2.3 per 100,000 women), Western Africa (2.4 per 100,000 women), and Eastern Africa (2.6 per 100,000 women).

The global mortality rate of endometrial cancer was 1.8 per 100,000 women in 2020, resulting in about 97,370 deaths. The mortality rate reflects the number of deaths from a disease relative to the population size. The global mortality rate of endometrial cancer is lower than the global incidence rate, indicating that endometrial cancer has a relatively high survival rate compared to other cancers.

However, the mortality rate also varies by region, with some regions having higher or lower rates than others. The highest mortality rates of endometrial cancer in 2020 were found in the Caribbean (4.6 per 100,000 women), Melanesia (4.1 per 100,000 women), and Eastern Europe (3.9 per 100,000 women). The lowest mortality rates of endometrial cancer in 2020 were found in Eastern Africa (0.8 per 100,000 women), Southern Africa (0.9 per 100,000 women), and Western Africa (1.0 per 100,000 women).

The global prevalence of endometrial cancer is the proportion of women who have ever been diagnosed with endometrial cancer and are still alive at a given point in time. The global prevalence of endometrial cancer in 2020 was estimated to be 1,153,000 cases or 0.3% of the female population. The prevalence of endometrial cancer depends on the incidence, mortality, and survival rates of the disease, as well as the population size and age structure. The prevalence of endometrial cancer is higher in regions with higher incidence and survival rates and lower in regions with lower incidence and survival rates.

US statistics and prevalence

Endometrial cancer is the most common female reproductive organ cancer in the United States and the fourth most common cancer among women. According to the American Cancer Society, there will be around 67,880 new cases of uterine cancer, including endometrial cancers and uterine sarcomas, in 2024.

Uterine sarcomas are rare types of uterine cancer that originate in the muscle or connective tissue of the uterus. Approximately 10% of uterine cancers are sarcomas. It is estimated that about 13,250 women will lose their lives to uterine cancer in 2024. However, the actual numbers for endometrial cancer cases and deaths are slightly lower than these estimates since the mentioned figures also include uterine sarcomas.

The US incidence rate of endometrial cancer was 21.4 per 100,000 women in 2017, the most recent year for which data are available. The US incidence rate of endometrial cancer is higher than the global average and ranks ninth among the countries with the highest rates of endometrial cancer. The US incidence rate of endometrial cancer has been increasing over the past decade by about 1% per year in White women and 2% to 3% per year in women of all other racial and ethnic groups.

This may be due to several factors, such as the rising rates of obesity, diabetes, and estrogen exposure, which are known to increase the risk of endometrial cancer. Other factors, such as environmental exposures, lifestyle habits, and access to health care, may also play a role.

The US mortality rate of endometrial cancer was 4.4 per 100,000 women in 2017. The US mortality rate of endometrial cancer is lower than the global average and ranks 28th among the countries with the highest rates of endometrial cancer. The US mortality rate of endometrial cancer is one of the few cancers with increasing mortality; since the mid-2000s, the death rate has risen by 1.7% per year.

This may be due to the increasing incidence of endometrial cancer as well as the challenges in detecting and treating advanced or recurrent cases. Black women are more likely to die from endometrial cancer than White women, which may reflect the disparities in risk factors, screening, diagnosis, treatment, and follow-up care.

The US prevalence of endometrial cancer is the proportion of women who have ever been diagnosed with endometrial cancer and are still alive at a given point in time. The US prevalence of endometrial cancer in 2018 was estimated to be 635,000 cases or 0.4% of the female population. The US prevalence of endometrial cancer is higher than the global average and ranks fifth among the countries with the highest prevalence of endometrial cancer.

The prevalence of endometrial cancer in the US depends on the incidence, mortality, and survival rates of the disease, as well as the population size and age structure. The prevalence of endometrial cancer in the US is higher in regions with higher incidence and survival rates and lower in regions with lower incidence and survival rates.

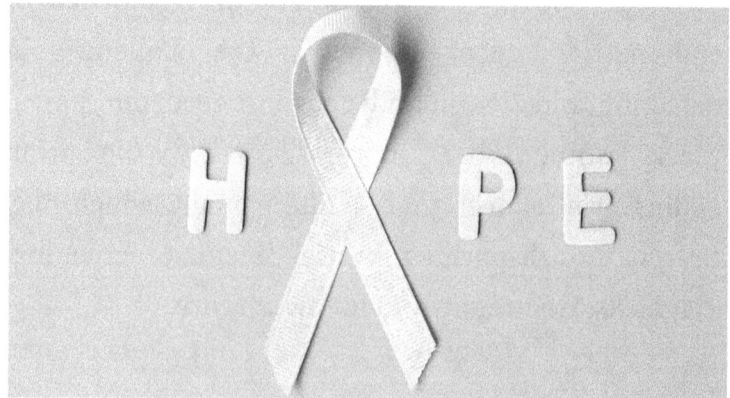

Chapter 2

Causes and Risk Factors

Known Causes of Endometrial Cancer

The exact cause of endometrial cancer is unknown. However, it is believed to be related to changes in the balance of hormones in the body, especially estrogen and progesterone. These hormones affect the growth and shedding of the endometrium, the lining of the uterus.

With too much estrogen and insufficient progesterone, the endometrium may grow too thick and not shed properly. This can lead to the accumulation of abnormal cells that can become cancerous over time.

Some of the factors that can increase the levels of estrogen or decrease the levels of progesterone in the body are:

- **Obesity:** Fat tissue can produce estrogen, so having more fat tissue can increase the estrogen levels in the body.
- **Hormone therapy:** Taking estrogen alone after menopause can increase the risk of endometrial cancer unless it is balanced by progesterone or progestin (a synthetic form of progesterone). Taking tamoxifen, a drug used to treat breast cancer can also increase the risk of endometrial cancer because it acts like estrogen on the endometrium.
- **Ovarian tumors:** Some tumors of the ovaries, such as granulosa cell tumors, can produce estrogen and increase the estrogen levels in the body.
- **Menstrual history:** Having more menstrual cycles over a lifetime can increase the exposure of the endometrium to estrogen. This can happen if a woman starts menstruating at an early age (before 12), has a

late menopause (after 55), or has never been pregnant.

- **Genetic conditions:** Some inherited conditions, such as Lynch syndrome or Cowden syndrome, can increase the risk of endometrial cancer because they cause defects in the genes that repair DNA damage in the cells. This can lead to the accumulation of mutations that can cause cancer.

- **Polycystic Ovary Syndrome (PCOS):** Women with PCOS have a hormonal imbalance, including higher estrogen levels that boost endometrial cancer odds. Irregular periods also mean less frequent sloughing of the excess lining.

These factors do not cause endometrial cancer by themselves, but they can increase the likelihood of developing it. Identifying and understanding these contributory factors is key to recognizing personal risk and undergoing appropriate screening to enable early detection.

Risk Factors and Their Impact

The risk factor increases the chance of developing a disease like cancer. Different cancers have different risk factors; some are more important than others. Having a risk factor does not mean that a person will get the disease, and not having a risk factor does not mean that a person will not. Many people with risk factors never develop endometrial cancer, and some people with endometrial cancer have no known risk factors.

In this section, we will discuss some of the major risk factors for endometrial cancer and how they affect the likelihood and severity of the disease. We will also provide tips on reducing or managing these risk factors and lowering the risk of endometrial cancer.

Obesity

Obesity is one of the strongest and most modifiable risk factors for endometrial cancer. Obesity is having a body mass index (BMI) of 30 or higher. BMI is a measure of body fat based on height and weight. Your BMI is found using our body mass index (BMI) calculator.

Obesity increases the risk of endometrial cancer by affecting the levels of hormones in the body, especially estrogen and insulin. Estrogen is a female hormone that stimulates the endometrium's growth, the uterus's lining. Insulin is a hormone that regulates blood sugar levels and promotes fat storage. Both hormones can promote the growth and survival of abnormal cells that can become cancerous.

Obesity can increase the levels of estrogen and insulin in the body in several ways:

- Fat tissue can produce estrogen from other hormones, such as androgens. More fat tissue can increase the amount of estrogen in the body, especially after menopause, when the ovaries stop producing estrogen.
- Obesity can cause insulin resistance, a condition where the cells do not respond well to insulin, and the body needs more insulin to keep blood sugar levels normal. High insulin levels can stimulate the production of estrogen and androgens by the ovaries and adrenal glands and reduce the production of

sex hormone-binding globulin (SHBG). This protein binds to and inactivates estrogen and androgens in the blood. This can result in higher levels of free or active hormones in the body.

- Obesity can cause chronic inflammation, in which the immune system is constantly activated and produces substances that can damage the cells and the DNA. Inflammation can also stimulate the production of estrogen and insulin and interfere with their normal functions.

Studies have shown that obesity can increase the risk of endometrial cancer by 2 to 4 times, depending on the degree of obesity. Obesity can also increase the risk of more aggressive types of endometrial cancer, such as serous and clear cell carcinomas, which are more likely to spread and recur. Obesity can also affect the diagnosis and treatment of endometrial cancer, as obese women may have more difficulty undergoing pelvic exams, imaging tests, biopsies, surgeries, and radiation therapy.

The impact of obesity on endometrial cancer risk can be reduced by losing weight and maintaining a healthy weight. Weight loss can lower estrogen, insulin, and inflammation levels in the body and improve hormonal balance and immune function. Weight loss can also improve the symptoms and outcomes of endometrial cancer treatment and reduce the risk of recurrence and other health problems.

Hormone therapy

Hormone therapy uses medications that contain hormones or affect the levels of hormones in the body. Hormone therapy can be used for various purposes, such as treating menopausal symptoms, preventing osteoporosis, or treating certain cancers. Hormone therapy can affect the risk of endometrial cancer, depending on the type, dose, duration, and timing of the therapy.

The main types of hormone therapy that can affect the risk of endometrial cancer are:

- **Estrogen therapy:** The use of estrogen alone, without progesterone or progestin (a synthetic form of progesterone), to treat menopausal symptoms such as hot flashes, night sweats, vaginal dryness, and mood swings. Estrogen therapy can increase the risk of endometrial cancer by stimulating the growth of the endometrium without the counterbalancing effect of progesterone or progestin. The risk of endometrial cancer increases with the dose and duration of estrogen therapy and decreases after stopping the therapy.

- **Tamoxifen:** A drug that blocks the action of estrogen on breast cancer cells but acts like estrogen on the endometrium. Tamoxifen is used to treat and prevent breast cancer in women who have estrogen receptor-positive (ER+) tumors. Tamoxifen can increase the risk of endometrial cancer by stimulating the growth of the endometrium, especially in postmenopausal women. The risk of endometrial cancer increases with the dose and duration of tamoxifen and decreases after stopping the drug.

- **Combined hormone therapy:** The use of estrogen plus progesterone or progestin to treat menopausal symptoms and prevent osteoporosis. Combined hormone therapy can lower the risk of endometrial cancer by preventing the overgrowth of the endometrium, as long as the progesterone or the progestin is taken for at least 10 to 14 days each month. However, combined hormone therapy can increase the risk of other health problems, such as breast cancer, heart disease, stroke, and blood clots.

The impact of hormone therapy on endometrial cancer risk can be reduced by using the lowest effective dose for the shortest possible time and by monitoring the endometrium regularly with pelvic exams, ultrasounds, and biopsies. It is also important to discuss the benefits and risks of hormone therapy with your doctor and to consider other options for treating menopausal symptoms, preventing osteoporosis, or treating breast cancer, such as non-hormonal medications, lifestyle changes, or alternative therapies.

Ovarian tumors

Ovarian tumors are abnormal growths that develop in the ovaries, the pair of organs that produce eggs and hormones in women. Ovarian tumors can be benign (non-cancerous) or malignant (cancerous) and can affect the levels of hormones in the body, especially estrogen. Some of the ovarian tumors that can increase the risk of endometrial cancer are:

- **Granulosa cell tumors:** These are rare types of ovarian cancer that arise from the granulosa cells, which are the cells that surround the eggs and produce estrogen. Granulosa cell tumors can produce large amounts of estrogen, which can stimulate the growth of the endometrium and increase the risk of endometrial cancer. Granulosa cell tumors can occur at any age but are more common in postmenopausal women.

- **Polycystic ovarian syndrome (PCOS):** This is a common condition that affects the balance of hormones in the body, causing irregular periods, excess hair growth, acne, weight gain, and infertility. PCOS is caused by the overproduction of androgens (male hormones) by the ovaries, which can interfere with the normal development and release of eggs. PCOS can also cause insulin resistance, a condition where the cells do not respond well to insulin, and the body needs more insulin to keep the blood sugar levels normal. PCOS can increase the risk of endometrial cancer by reducing the levels of progesterone and increasing the levels of estrogen and insulin in the body. This can result in the overgrowth of the endometrium and the accumulation of abnormal cells that can become cancerous. PCOS can occur at any age but is more common in women of reproductive age.

The impact of ovarian tumors on endometrial cancer risk can be reduced by treating the tumors and restoring the average hormonal balance. The treatment of ovarian tumors depends on the type, size, location, and stage of the tumor, as well as the age, health, and fertility of the patient.

Menstrual history

Menstrual history refers to the pattern and duration of a woman's menstrual cycles, which are the monthly changes in the body that prepare for a possible pregnancy. Menstrual history can affect the risk of endometrial cancer by influencing the exposure of the endometrium to estrogen and progesterone. Some of the aspects of menstrual history that can increase the risk of endometrial cancer are:

- **Early menarche:** This is the age when a girl has her first menstrual period. The average age of menarche in the US is 12.5 years, but it can vary from 8 to 16 years. Having an early menarche can increase the risk of endometrial cancer by increasing the number of menstrual cycles and the exposure of the endometrium to estrogen over a lifetime. Studies have shown that for every year earlier that menarche occurs, the risk of endometrial cancer increases by 2% to 4%.

- **Late menopause:** This is the age when a woman has her last menstrual period. The average age of menopause in the US is 51 years, but it can vary from 40 to 60 years. Having a late menopause can increase the risk of endometrial cancer by increasing the number of menstrual cycles and the exposure of the endometrium to estrogen over a lifetime. Studies have shown that every year after menopause occurs, the risk of endometrial cancer increases by 2% to 3%.

- **Never being pregnant:** This is the condition of never having a full-term pregnancy. Pregnancy can lower the risk of endometrial cancer by reducing the number of menstrual cycles and the exposure of the endometrium to estrogen. Pregnancy can also cause changes in the endometrium that make it less likely to develop cancer. Studies have shown that women who have never been pregnant have a 2–3 times higher risk of endometrial cancer than women who have had at least one full-term pregnancy.

- **Infertility:** This is the condition of not being able to get pregnant after trying for at least a year. Infertility can increase the risk of endometrial cancer by affecting the levels of hormones in the body, especially estrogen and progesterone. Various factors, such as ovulation problems, polycystic ovarian syndrome, endometriosis, pelvic inflammatory disease, or tubal blockage, can cause infertility. Some of these factors can also increase the risk of endometrial cancer by themselves. Infertility can also prevent pregnancy, which can lower the risk of endometrial cancer.

The impact of menstrual history on endometrial cancer risk can be reduced by modifying some of the factors that affect hormonal balance and endometrial growth. For example, taking oral contraceptives (birth control pills) can lower the risk of endometrial cancer by suppressing ovulation and reducing the levels of estrogen and progesterone in the body. Oral contraceptives can also regulate the menstrual cycles and prevent abnormal bleeding.

Studies have shown that women who use oral contraceptives have a 30% to 50% lower risk of endometrial cancer than women who do not use them, and the protective effect lasts for at least 10 years after stopping the use. However, oral contraceptives can also have some side effects and risks, such as blood clots, stroke, and breast cancer, so they should be used with caution and under medical supervision.

Chapter 3

Recognizing the Symptoms

Common Symptoms of Endometrial Cancer

One of the most important steps in preventing and treating endometrial cancer is to recognize its symptoms and seek medical attention as soon as possible. Endometrial cancer can cause various signs and symptoms, depending on the stage and type of the cancer as well as the individual characteristics of the patient. However, some symptoms are more common and more likely to indicate endometrial cancer than others. These common symptoms are:

- **Abnormal vaginal bleeding or discharge:** This is the most common symptom of endometrial cancer, and it occurs in about 90% of cases. Abnormal bleeding or discharge can include bleeding between periods, bleeding after menopause, bleeding after sexual intercourse, spotting, or a watery or blood-tinged discharge. The bleeding or discharge may be light or heavy, varying in color, consistency, and odor. Any abnormal vaginal bleeding or discharge should be reported to a doctor, especially if it persists or worsens.

- **Pelvic pain or pressure:** This is a less common symptom of endometrial cancer, and it occurs in about 10% to 20% of cases. Pelvic pain or pressure can include cramping, aching, or discomfort in the lower abdomen, back, or legs. The pain or pressure may be constant or intermittent, varying in intensity and location. The growth of the tumor may cause pelvic pain or pressure, the invasion of the surrounding tissues, or the spread of the cancer to other organs. A doctor should evaluate pelvic pain or pressure that is severe, persistent, or unexplained.

- **Difficulty urinating or defecating:** This is a rare symptom of endometrial cancer, and it occurs in less than 5% of cases. Difficulty urinating or defecating can include pain, burning, urgency, frequency, incontinence, or obstruction of the urine or stool. Difficulty urinating or defecating may be caused by the compression or invasion of the bladder, ureters, rectum, or anus by the tumor or the cancer cells. Difficulty urinating or defecating that is severe, persistent, or unexplained should be checked by a doctor.

These are some of the common symptoms of endometrial cancer, but they are not specific to this disease. Other conditions, such as infections, hormonal changes, fibroids, polyps, or other cancers, may also cause them.

When to Seek Medical Attention

Endometrial cancer can be treated successfully if it is detected early, but it can also cause serious complications and death if it is left untreated or diagnosed late. Knowing when to seek medical evaluation for potential endometrial cancer symptoms can make a crucial difference in early diagnosis and more positive outcomes. Do not ignore worrisome changes.

Contact your doctor promptly if you experience:

- Vaginal bleeding after menopause. Any postmenopausal bleeding warrants immediate medical attention to rule out endometrial cancer. About 90% of women diagnosed with endometrial cancer have reported vaginal bleeding after menopause as a symptom. It should not be considered normal or harmless.
- Heavy or prolonged menstrual bleeding before menopause. Bleeding lasting over 7 days or soaking through a pad or tampon every hour for several hours merits evaluation.
- Pelvic pain that persists. Intermittent mild pelvic pain may occur during the menstrual cycle. However, constant pelvic pain or pressure that lasts for weeks requires medical assessment. Pain radiating to the thighs or lower back is also of concern.

- Unexplained weight loss. Losing weight without trying could reflect hormonal changes from endometrial cancer. Appetite loss and change in energy levels may accompany weight loss.
- Persistent unusual discharge. Watery, blood-tinged, or foul-smelling discharge that differs from your regular secretions should be examined.
- Painful intercourse. Seek care if you regularly experience pain during sex that did not previously occur.
- Trouble urinating. Straining, frequent urination, inability to empty the bladder, and other urinary symptoms warrant evaluation. Blood in urine requires immediate attention.

Even if symptoms seem minor at first, do not delay seeking care. Symptoms that persist for 2-3 weeks without improvement necessitate making an appointment. The sooner any endometrial abnormalities can be detected, the better.

Be prepared to share details on your symptoms, menstrual cycle, medical history, and family history with your doctor. They will determine the next steps, which may include an ultrasound, biopsy, or other tests to reach a diagnosis and develop an appropriate treatment plan.

The earlier you seek medical attention for endometrial cancer, the better your chances of survival and recovery. Do not delay or hesitate to contact your doctor if you have any concerns or questions about your health and well-being.

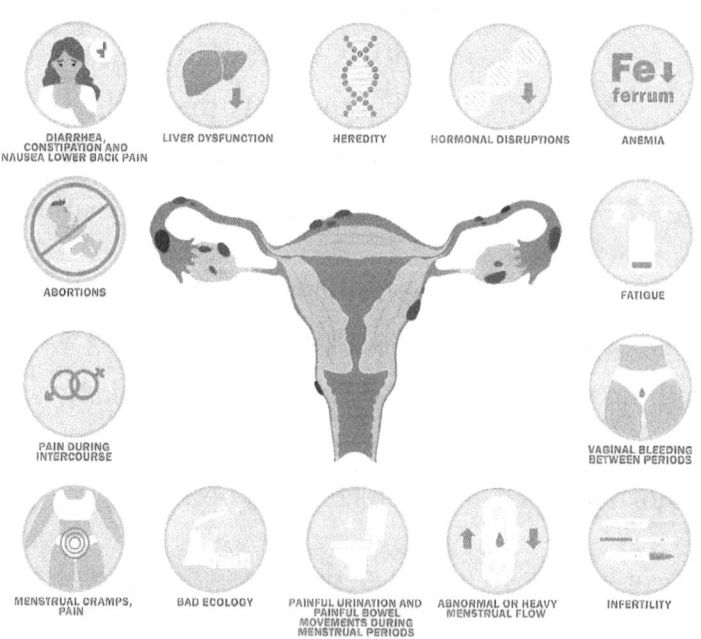

SYMPTOMS OF ENDOMETRIOSIS

DIARRHEA, CONSTIPATION AND NAUSEA LOWER BACK PAIN

LIVER DYSFUNCTION

HEREDITY

HORMONAL DISRUPTIONS

ANEMIA

ABORTIONS

FATIGUE

PAIN DURING INTERCOURSE

VAGINAL BLEEDING BETWEEN PERIODS

MENSTRUAL CRAMPS, PAIN

BAD ECOLOGY

PAINFUL URINATION AND PAINFUL BOWEL MOVEMENTS DURING MENSTRUAL PERIODS

ABNORMAL OR HEAVY MENSTRUAL FLOW

INFERTILITY

Chapter 4

Diagnosis and Testing of Endometrial Cancer

Diagnostic Tests and Procedures

In this section, we will discuss the diagnostic tests and procedures used to detect and confirm endometrial cancer and determine its stage, grade, type, and location. These tests and procedures can help doctors plan the best treatment and predict the outcome for each patient. Some of the diagnostic tests and procedures for endometrial cancer are:

- **Pelvic exam:** A pelvic exam is a physical examination of the reproductive organs. It is often done during a regular checkup; however, it may be needed if you have symptoms of endometrial cancer, such as abnormal vaginal bleeding or discharge, pelvic pain or pressure, or difficulty urinating or defecating. During the exam, a doctor or a nurse carefully inspects the outer genitals, inserts two fingers into the vagina and presses on the abdomen to feel the uterus and ovaries, and inserts a device called a speculum into the vagina to look for signs of cancer or other problems in the cervix and the endometrium.

- **Ultrasound:** Ultrasound is an imaging test that uses sound waves to create pictures of the inside of the body. It can help doctors see the size, shape, and structure of the uterus, ovaries, and fallopian tubes and look for any masses or abnormalities. Two types of ultrasound can be used for endometrial cancer: transvaginal ultrasound and saline infusion sonogram. A transvaginal ultrasound involves inserting a wand-like device called a transducer into the vagina, which emits sound waves and picks up the echoes as they bounce off the organs. A saline infusion sonogram involves injecting salt water (saline) into the uterus before the ultrasound, which helps the doctors see the endometrial lining more clearly.

- **Endometrial biopsy:** An endometrial biopsy is a procedure that involves removing a small sample of tissue from the endometrium, the lining of the uterus. The sample is then sent to a lab and examined under a microscope for cancer cells. An endometrial biopsy can be done in a doctor's office using a thin, flexible tube called a pipelle that is inserted through the cervix and into the uterus. The tube is then moved back and forth to collect the tissue. An endometrial biopsy can cause some cramping, bleeding, or spotting, but it is usually well tolerated by most women.

- **Dilation and curettage (D&C):** A D&C is a procedure that involves scraping or suctioning tissue from the inside of the uterus. It is usually done in a hospital or a clinic, under general or local anesthesia. A D&C may be needed if an endometrial biopsy does not provide enough tissue for testing or if the biopsy results are unclear. A D&C can also help treat some conditions that cause abnormal bleeding, such as polyps or fibroids. A D&C can cause some bleeding, cramping, or discomfort, but it is usually safe and effective.

- **Hysteroscopy:** A hysteroscopy is a procedure that involves using a thin, flexible, lighted tube called a hysteroscope to examine the inside of the uterus. The hysteroscope is inserted through the vagina and cervix and into the uterus, and a lens on the hysteroscope allows the doctor to see the endometrium and the uterine cavity. A hysteroscopy can help diagnose endometrial cancer, as well as other conditions that affect the uterus, such as polyps, fibroids, or adhesions. A hysteroscopy can also perform a biopsy or a D&C if needed. A hysteroscopy can cause some bleeding, cramping, or infection, but it is usually safe and well tolerated by most women.

- **Imaging tests:** Imaging tests use different methods to create pictures of the inside of the body. They can help doctors see the extent and spread of endometrial cancer and plan the best treatment for each patient. Some of the imaging tests that can be used for endometrial cancer are chest X-ray, computed tomography (CT) scan, magnetic resonance imaging (MRI) scan, and positron emission tomography (PET) scan. A chest X-ray uses X-rays to create pictures of the chest and lungs and can help detect if endometrial cancer has spread to these organs. A CT scan uses X-rays and a computer to create detailed cross-sectional images of the body, and it can help show the size and location of endometrial cancer and if it has spread to nearby organs or lymph nodes.

MRI scans use radio waves and a powerful magnet to create detailed body images. It can help show the depth and extent of endometrial cancer and if it has invaded the muscle layer of the uterus or the surrounding tissues. A PET scan uses a radioactive substance called a tracer that is injected into the blood and a special camera to create images of the body. It can help show how active the endometrial cancer cells are and if they have spread to distant organs or lymph nodes. These imaging tests can cause discomfort, allergic reactions, or radiation exposure, but they are usually safe and accurate.

Understanding Your Diagnosis

After undergoing the diagnostic tests and procedures for endometrial cancer, your doctor will explain the results and what they mean for your condition and treatment. Understanding your diagnosis can help you make informed decisions about your health and well-being. In this subchapter, we will discuss some of the key aspects of your diagnosis, such as the stage, grade, type, and location of your endometrial cancer and how they affect your prognosis and treatment options.

Stage

The stage of endometrial cancer describes how far the cancer has spread from its original site in the endometrium, the lining of the uterus. The stage of endometrial cancer is determined by the results of the biopsy, imaging tests, and sometimes surgery. The stage of endometrial cancer is one of the most important factors that affect your prognosis and treatment plan.

The most common system used to stage endometrial cancer is the TNM system, which stands for tumor, node, and metastasis. The TNM system assigns a number or a letter to each of the three categories based on the tumor's size and extent, the lymph nodes' involvement, and the cancer's spread to other parts of the body. The TNM system also combines these categories into four main stages, from stage I to stage IV, with some sub-stages. The higher the stage, the more advanced the cancer.

The following is a summary of the TNM system and the stages of endometrial cancer:

- **Tumor (T):** The tumor category describes the size and extent of the primary tumor in the uterus. It is divided into four sub-categories, from T1 to T4, with some further subdivisions. The higher the T number, the larger or deeper the tumor.
  - ○ **T1:** The tumor is confined to the endometrium or the inner half of the muscle layer of the uterus (myometrium). It is further divided into:

1. **T1a:** The tumor is limited to the endometrium or invades less than half of the myometrium.
2. **T1b:** The tumor invades more than half of the myometrium.

○ **T2:** The tumor invades the outer half of the myometrium but does not reach the uterus's (serosa) outer surface or the tissues around the uterus (adnexa).

○ **T3:** The tumor invades the serosa, the adnexa, or both. It is further divided into:

   1. **T3a:** The tumor invades the uterus's outer layer, serosa.
   2. **T3b:** The tumor invades the adnexa, the tissues around the uterus, such as the ovaries, fallopian tubes, or ligaments.

○ **T4:** The tumor invades the bladder, the rectum, or both or grows outside the pelvis.

- **<u>Node (N):</u>** The node category describes the involvement of the regional lymph nodes. These small, bean-shaped organs filter and drain lymph fluid and help fight infections and diseases. The lymph nodes near the uterus are called the pelvic and para-aortic lymph nodes. The node category is divided into two sub-categories, N0 and N1, with some further subdivisions. The higher the N number, the more lymph nodes are affected.

- o **N0:** No regional lymph nodes are involved.
- o **N1:** Regional lymph nodes are involved. It is further divided into:
    1. **N1a:** Only pelvic lymph nodes are involved.
    2. **N1b:** Only para-aortic lymph nodes are involved.
    3. **N1c:** Both pelvic and para-aortic lymph nodes are involved.

- **Metastasis (M):** The metastasis category describes the spread of the cancer to distant parts of the body, such as the lungs, liver, bones, or brain. The metastasis category is divided into two sub-categories, M0 and M1.

The higher the M number, the more distant organs are affected.

- ○ **M0:** No distant metastasis is found.
- ○ **M1:** Distant metastasis is found.

The TNM categories are then combined into four main stages, from stage I to stage IV, with some sub-stages. The following is a summary of the stages of endometrial cancer and their definitions:

- **Stage I:** The cancer is confined to the uterus. It is further divided into:
  - ○ **Stage IA:** The cancer is limited to the endometrium or invades less than half of the myometrium, and no lymph nodes are involved (T1a N0 M0).
  - ○ **Stage IB:** The cancer invades more than half of the myometrium, and no lymph nodes are involved (T1b N0 M0).

- **Stage II:** The cancer invades the outer half of the myometrium but does not reach the serosa, the adnexa, or the lymph nodes (T2 N0 M0).

- **Stage III:** The cancer invades the serosa, the adnexa, the lymph nodes, or all of them but does not spread to distant organs. It is further divided into:
  - ○ **Stage IIIA:** The cancer invades the serosa, and no lymph nodes are involved (T3a N0 M0).
  - ○ **Stage IIIB:** The cancer invades the adnexa, and no lymph nodes are involved (T3b N0 M0).
  - ○ **Stage IIIC:** The cancer invades the pelvic and para-aortic lymph nodes, regardless of the extent of the tumor in the uterus (T1-T3 N1 M0). It is further divided into:
    1. **Stage IIIC1:** The cancer invades only the pelvic lymph nodes (T1-T3 N1a M0).
    2. **Stage IIIC2:** The cancer invades the para-aortic lymph nodes, with or without pelvic lymph node involvement (T1-T3 N1b-N1c M0).

- **Stage IV:** The cancer invades the bladder, the rectum, or both, grows outside the pelvis, or spreads to distant organs. It is further divided into:
  - **Stage IVA:** The cancer invades the bladder, the rectum, or both (T4 N0-N1 M0).
  - **Stage IVB:** The cancer grows outside the pelvis and spreads to distant organs (Any T Any N M1).

The stage of endometrial cancer can affect your prognosis and treatment options. Generally, the earlier the stage, the better the prognosis and the more treatment options available. The later the stage, the worse the prognosis and the fewer available treatment options.

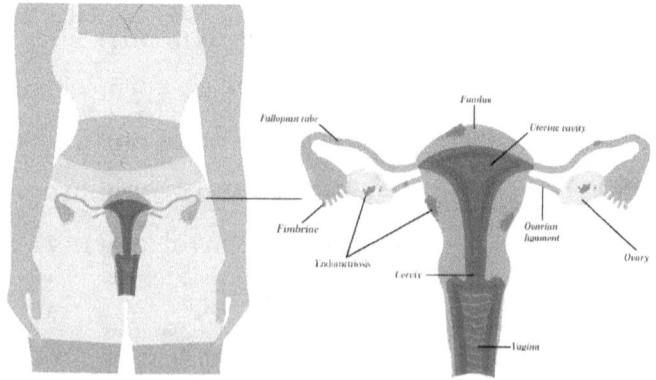

Chapter 5

Treatment Options

Overview of Available Treatment Options

The treatment options for endometrial cancer depend on several factors, such as the stage, grade, type, and location of the cancer, as well as the age, health, and preferences of the patient. The main goals of treatment are to remove the cancer, prevent it from spreading or coming back, and relieve the symptoms and side effects. The main treatment options for endometrial cancer are:

- Surgery is the first and most common treatment for endometrial cancer. It involves removing the uterus, cervix, fallopian tubes, and ovaries, which is called a total hysterectomy and bilateral salpingo-oophorectomy (TH/BSO). Sometimes, the lymph nodes near the uterus are also removed and tested for cancer spread, which is called a pelvic and para-aortic lymph node dissection (LND) or sampling. Surgery can cure endometrial cancer if it is confined to the uterus. However, it also means that the patient can no longer get pregnant or have menstrual periods. Surgery may also cause some complications, such as bleeding, infection, or damage to nearby organs.

- Radiation therapy uses high-energy rays or particles to kill cancer cells or stop them from growing. It can be given externally, by a machine that aims the radiation at the pelvis, or internally, by placing radioactive sources inside the vagina or the uterus, which is called brachytherapy. Radiation therapy can be used before surgery to shrink the tumor, after surgery to kill any remaining cancer cells, or instead of surgery for patients who cannot have surgery or do not want to have surgery. Radiation therapy can also help relieve the symptoms of advanced or recurrent endometrial cancer, such as bleeding or pain. Radiation therapy may cause some side effects, such as skin irritation, fatigue, nausea, diarrhea, or bladder problems.

- Chemotherapy uses drugs to kill or stop cancer cells from dividing. It can be given by mouth, injection, or infusion into a vein. Chemotherapy can be used after surgery to lower the risk of recurrence, especially for patients with high-risk or advanced endometrial cancer. It can also be used for patients who cannot have surgery or radiation therapy or for patients whose cancer has spread to distant organs or come back after initial treatment. Chemotherapy may cause some side effects, such as hair loss, mouth sores, loss of appetite, vomiting, low blood cell counts, or nerve damage.

- Hormone therapy uses drugs to block or lower the levels of hormones, such as estrogen and progesterone, that can stimulate the growth of some types of endometrial cancer. It can be given by mouth, by injection, or by implant. Hormone therapy can be used before surgery to shrink the tumor, especially for young patients who want to preserve their fertility, or after surgery to lower the risk of recurrence, especially for patients with low-risk or early-stage endometrial cancer. It can also be used for patients who cannot have surgery, radiation therapy, or chemotherapy or for patients whose cancer has spread to distant organs or come back after initial treatment. Hormone therapy may cause some side effects, such as weight gain, fluid retention, hot flashes, vaginal dryness, or mood changes.

- Targeted therapy uses drugs to target specific molecules or pathways involved in cancer cells' growth and survival. It can be given by mouth, injection, or infusion into a vein. Targeted therapy can be used for patients with advanced or recurrent endometrial cancer that has a certain genetic mutation or biomarker, such as mismatch repair deficiency (dMMR), microsatellite instability-high (MSI-H), or programmed death-ligand 1 (PD-L1). Targeted therapy may work better than chemotherapy or hormone therapy for some patients. It may cause fewer or different side effects, such as skin rash, diarrhea, or liver problems.

These are some of the main treatment options for endometrial cancer, but they are not the only ones. Other treatment options may include immunotherapy, which uses drugs to boost the immune system to fight cancer, or clinical trials, which are research studies that test new or experimental treatments. The best treatment option for each patient depends on their situation and preferences.

Surgery

Surgery is the main treatment option for most cases of endometrial cancer. It involves removing the uterus and other reproductive organs, as well as the lymph nodes near the uterus, to get rid of the cancer and prevent it from spreading. The type and extent of surgery depend on the stage, grade, type, and location of the cancer, as well as the patient's age, health, and preferences. Here, we will discuss the different types of surgery for endometrial cancer and their benefits and risks.

Hysterectomy

A hysterectomy is an operation that removes the uterus and cervix. It is the most common surgery for endometrial cancer, and it can cure the cancer if it is confined to the uterus. A hysterectomy can be done differently, depending on the situation and the surgeon'ssurgeon's preference. The main types of hysterectomy are:

- **Abdominal hysterectomy:** The uterus and cervix are removed through a large cut (incision) in the lower abdomen (belly). This type of hysterectomy allows the surgeon to see and remove the uterus and other organs more easily. However, it also has a longer recovery time and more complications than other types of hysterectomy.

- **Vaginal hysterectomy:** The uterus and cervix are removed through the vagina without making any incisions in the abdomen. This type of hysterectomy has a shorter recovery time and fewer complications than an abdominal hysterectomy. However, it may not be suitable for patients with large tumors or advanced cancer, as the surgeon has less access and visibility to the pelvic organs.

- **Laparoscopic hysterectomy:** The uterus and cervix are removed through several small incisions in the abdomen using a thin, flexible tube with a light camera (laparoscope) and special instruments. This type of hysterectomy has the advantages of both an abdominal and a vaginal hysterectomy, as it allows the surgeon to see and remove the uterus and other organs more precisely while also having a shorter recovery time and fewer complications than an abdominal hysterectomy.

A hysterectomy can be either simple or radical, depending on how much of the surrounding tissues and organs are removed along with the uterus and cervix. A simple hysterectomy removes only the uterus and cervix. In contrast, a radical hysterectomy removes the entire uterus, the tissues next to the uterus (parametrium and uterosacral ligaments), and the upper part of the vagina (next to the cervix).

A radical hysterectomy is usually done for patients with advanced or aggressive endometrial cancer, as it can remove more cancer cells and lower the risk of recurrence. A hysterectomy can also be combined with other procedures, such as:

- **Bilateral salpingo-oophorectomy (BSO):** Removing both fallopian tubes and ovaries. This is usually done for most patients with endometrial cancer, as it can lower the levels of hormones that can stimulate the growth of some types of endometrial cancer and also prevent ovarian cancer, which is another common cancer of the female reproductive organs.

- **Lymph node dissection or sampling:** The removal of some or all of the lymph nodes in the pelvis and around the aorta, the small, bean-shaped organs that filter and drain lymph fluid and help fight infections and diseases. This is done to check if the cancer has spread to the lymph nodes and to remove any cancer cells that may be in them. Lymph node dissection removes more lymph nodes than lymph node sampling. However, it also has a higher risk of complications, such as lymphedema (swelling of the legs due to fluid buildup).

- **Pelvic washings:** The collection of fluid from the pelvis is then sent to a lab and examined for cancer cells. This is done to check if the cancer has spread to the pelvic cavity and to remove any cancer cells that may be in the fluid.

- **Omentectomy:** The removal of the omentum, a layer of fatty tissue covering and protecting the abdominal organs. This is done to check if the cancer has spread to the omentum and to remove any cancer cells that may be in it.

- **Peritoneal biopsies:** The removal of small tissue samples from the abdominal cavity's peritoneum lining. This is done to check if the cancer has spread to the peritoneum and to remove any cancer cells that may be in it.

The benefits of a hysterectomy for endometrial cancer are:

- It can cure the cancer if it is confined to the uterus or improve the chances of cure if it is combined with other treatments, such as radiation or chemotherapy.
- It can prevent the cancer from spreading or coming back or slow down its growth if it has already spread.
- It can relieve the symptoms of endometrial cancer, such as abnormal bleeding, pain, or pressure.

The risks of a hysterectomy for endometrial cancer are:

- It can cause complications, such as bleeding, infection, damage to nearby organs, blood clots, or anesthesia problems.
- It can cause side effects, such as menopause, infertility, sexual dysfunction, urinary incontinence, or bowel problems.
- It can affect the quality of life, such as the patient's emotional, social, and psychological well-being.

Debulking surgery

Debulking surgery is an operation that removes as much of the cancer as possible but not all of it. It is usually done for patients with advanced or recurrent endometrial cancer that has spread throughout the pelvis and abdomen (belly) and cannot be eradicated by surgery. Debulking surgery can be done in different ways, depending on the situation and the surgeon's preference. The main types of debulking surgery are:

- **Cytoreductive surgery:** The removal of the uterus, cervix, fallopian tubes, ovaries, lymph nodes, omentum, and any other organs or tissues that are affected by cancer, such as the bladder, rectum, liver, spleen, or intestines. This type of debulking surgery aims to remove as much of cancer as possible, leaving behind only small areas of cancer that cannot be seen or felt by the surgeon.

- **Palliative surgery:** The removal of only the parts of the cancer that are causing symptoms, such as bleeding, pain, or obstruction of the urine or stool. This type of debulking surgery aims to improve the quality of life of the patient but not to cure the cancer.

Debulking surgery can also be combined with other treatments, such as chemotherapy, radiation therapy, hormone therapy, or targeted therapy, to kill any remaining cancer cells and prevent or delay the cancer from growing or spreading. The benefits of debulking surgery for endometrial cancer are:

- It can improve the effectiveness of other treatments, such as chemotherapy, radiation therapy, hormone therapy, or targeted therapy, by reducing the cancer they have to target.
- It can improve the chances of survival or prolong the survival time by slowing down the growth and spread of the cancer.
- It can relieve the symptoms of endometrial cancer, such as bleeding, pain, or pressure.

The risks of debulking surgery for endometrial cancer are:

- It can cause complications, such as bleeding, infection, damage to nearby organs, blood clots, or anesthesia problems.
- It can cause side effects, such as menopause, infertility, sexual dysfunction, urinary incontinence, bowel problems, or nutritional problems.
- It can affect the quality of life, such as the patient's emotional, social, and psychological well-being.

Fertility-sparing surgery

Fertility-sparing surgery is an operation that preserves the ability to get pregnant in the future by removing only the part of the uterus that contains the cancer and leaving the rest of the uterus, cervix, fallopian tubes, and ovaries intact. It is also called a conservative surgery or a radical trachelectomy.

It is only done for young women with early-stage and low-grade endometrial cancer who still want to have children and who have no other risk factors or medical problems that would prevent them from having a successful pregnancy. Fertility-sparing surgery can be done in different ways, depending on the situation and the surgeon's preference. The main types of fertility-sparing surgery are:

- **Hysteroscopic resection:** The removal of the endometrium and the tumor through the vagina using a thin, flexible tube with a light and a camera (hysteroscope), and special instruments. This type of fertility-sparing surgery is suitable for patients with small and superficial tumors that do not invade the muscle layer of the uterus (myometrium).

- **Laparoscopic-assisted vaginal hysterectomy (LAVH):** The removal of the upper part of the uterus and the tumor through the vagina using a laparoscope and special instruments. The lower part of the uterus and the cervix are left in place. This type of fertility-sparing surgery is suitable for patients with more extensive or deeper tumors that invade the myometrium but not the cervix.

Fertility-sparing surgery can also be combined with other treatments, such as hormone therapy, to shrink the tumor before surgery or to lower the risk of recurrence after surgery. Hormone therapy uses drugs to block or lower the levels of hormones, such as estrogen and progesterone, that can stimulate the growth of some types of endometrial cancer. It can be given by mouth, by injection, or by implant.

The benefits of fertility-sparing surgery for endometrial cancer are:

- It can cure cancer if it is confined to the endometrium or improve the chances of a cure if it is combined with other treatments, such as hormone therapy.
- It can preserve the patient's fertility and menstrual function, allowing her to have children in the future.

The risks of fertility-sparing surgery for endometrial cancer are:

- It can cause complications, such as bleeding, infection, damage to nearby organs, or anesthesia problems.
- It can cause side effects, such as menstrual irregularities, ovarian cysts, or early menopause.

- It can increase the risk of recurrence, as some cancer cells may remain in the uterus or the cervix or develop later due to hormonal stimulation.
- It can affect the pregnancy outcomes, such as the risk of miscarriage, preterm delivery, or cesarean section.

Fertility-sparing surgery is not suitable for all patients with endometrial cancer, and it requires careful selection and close follow-up. It is only recommended for young women with early-stage and low-grade endometrial cancer who still want to have children and who have no other risk factors or medical problems that would prevent them from having a successful pregnancy.

It is also important to discuss the benefits and risks of fertility-sparing surgery with your doctor and to consider other options for preserving or achieving your fertility, such as egg or embryo freezing, surrogacy, or adoption.

Radiation Therapy

Radiation therapy is a treatment option for endometrial cancer that uses high-energy rays or particles to kill cancer cells or stop them from growing. It can be given in two ways: internally or externally. Here, we will discuss the different types of radiation therapy for endometrial cancer and their benefits and risks.

Internal radiation therapy

Internal radiation therapy, also called brachytherapy, involves placing radioactive sources inside the body near the tumor. The radiation mainly affects the area where the sources are placed and causes less damage to the surrounding healthy tissues. Internal radiation therapy can be used to treat endometrial cancer that is confined to the uterus or the upper part of the vagina or to boost the effect of external radiation therapy.

There are two types of internal radiation therapy for endometrial cancer: *low-dose rate (LDR)* and *high-dose rate (HDR)*. In LDR brachytherapy, the radioactive sources are left in place for several days, and the patient needs to stay in the hospital during the treatment. In HDR brachytherapy, the radioactive sources are inserted and removed within a few minutes, and the patient can go home after each treatment. HDR is more commonly used than LDR in the US.

The benefits of internal radiation therapy for endometrial cancer are:

- It can deliver a high dose of radiation to the tumor while sparing the nearby organs, such as the bladder and rectum, from too much radiation exposure.
- It can improve the chances of cure or prevent cancer from coming back, especially when combined with external radiation therapy or surgery.
- It can cause fewer side effects than external radiation therapy, such as skin irritation, fatigue, or nausea.

The risks of internal radiation therapy for endometrial cancer are:

- It can cause some discomfort, bleeding, or infection in the vagina, cervix, or uterus, where the radioactive sources are placed.
- It can cause some vaginal dryness, narrowing, or scarring, which may affect sexual function or intercourse.
- It can cause some temporary or permanent damage to the ovaries, which may affect fertility or hormone production.

External radiation therapy

External radiation therapy, also called external beam radiation therapy, involves using a machine that delivers radiation beams to the pelvis, where the tumor is located. The radiation beams can be shaped and adjusted to match the size and shape of the tumor, and to avoid the nearby healthy tissues. External radiation therapy can be used to treat endometrial cancer that has spread beyond the uterus or to lower the risk of recurrence after surgery.

There are different types of external radiation therapy for endometrial cancer, such as *3-dimensional conformal radiation therapy*

(3D-CRT), intensity modulated radiation therapy (IMRT), or image-guided radiation therapy (IGRT). These types of radiation therapy use advanced computer software and imaging techniques to deliver precise and accurate doses of radiation to the tumor while minimizing exposure to the surrounding normal tissues.

The benefits of external radiation therapy for endometrial cancer are:

- It can kill any cancer cells that may have spread to the pelvis or the lymph nodes, or that may have been left behind after surgery.
- It can improve the chances of survival, or prolong the survival time, by slowing down the growth and spread of the cancer.
- It can relieve the symptoms of endometrial cancer, such as bleeding, pain, or pressure.

The risks of external radiation therapy for endometrial cancer are:

- It can cause some skin irritation, redness, or peeling in the area where the radiation beams are aimed.

- It can cause some fatigue, nausea, diarrhea, or bladder problems, due to the radiation affecting the normal cells in the pelvis and abdomen.
- It can cause some vaginal dryness, narrowing, or scarring, which may affect sexual function or intercourse.
- It can cause some temporary or permanent damage to the ovaries, which may affect fertility or hormone production.

These are the main types of radiation therapy for endometrial cancer, but they are not the only ones. Other types of radiation therapy may include proton therapy, which uses protons instead of X-rays to deliver radiation, or stereotactic body radiation therapy (SBRT), which uses high doses of radiation in fewer sessions. The best type of radiation therapy for each patient depends on their individual situation and preferences.

Chemotherapy

Chemotherapy is a treatment option for endometrial cancer that uses drugs to kill cancer cells or stop them from dividing. It can be given by mouth, by injection, or by infusion into a vein. Chemotherapy can be used after surgery to lower the risk of recurrence, especially for patients with high-risk or advanced endometrial cancer.

It can also be used for patients who cannot have surgery or radiation therapy, or for patients whose cancer has spread to distant organs or come back after initial treatment. Chemotherapy may cause some side effects, such as hair loss, mouth sores, loss of appetite, vomiting, low blood cell counts, or nerve damage. Here, we will discuss the different types of chemotherapy drugs for endometrial cancer, and their benefits and risks.

Chemotherapy drugs

There are several chemotherapy drugs that can be used to treat endometrial cancer, either alone or in combination. The choice of drugs depends on the stage, grade, type, and location of the cancer, as well as the age, health, and preferences of the patient. Some of the most common chemotherapy drugs for endometrial cancer are:

- **Carboplatin:** A platinum-based drug that damages the DNA of cancer cells and prevents them from dividing. It is often combined with paclitaxel or docetaxel, which are drugs that interfere with the structure and function of microtubules, the components of the cell that help with cell division and movement.

- **Paclitaxel (Taxol ®):** A drug that interferes with the structure and function of microtubules, the components of the cell that help with cell division and movement. It is often combined with carboplatin, which is a platinum-based drug that damages the DNA of cancer cells and prevents them from dividing.

- **Docetaxel (Taxotere ®):** A drug that interferes with the structure and function of microtubules, the components of the cell that help with cell division and movement. It is often combined with carboplatin, which is a platinum-based drug that damages the DNA of cancer cells and prevents them from dividing.

- **Doxorubicin (Adriamycin ®) or liposomal doxorubicin (Doxil ®):** Drugs that belong to a group of drugs called anthracyclines, which work by inserting themselves into the DNA of cancer cells and preventing them from copying themselves. Liposomal doxorubicin is a form of doxorubicin that is enclosed in tiny fat particles (liposomes), which help deliver the drug to the tumor and reduce the damage to the heart, which is a common side effect of doxorubicin.

- **Cisplatin:** A platinum-based drug that damages the DNA of cancer cells and prevents them from dividing. It is often combined with doxorubicin, which is a drug that belongs to a group of drugs called anthracyclines, which work by inserting themselves into the DNA of cancer cells and preventing them from copying themselves.

- **Ifosfamide (Ifex ®):** A drug that belongs to a group of drugs called alkylating agents, which work by attaching chemical groups to the DNA of cancer cells and preventing them from copying themselves. It is often used for carcinosarcoma, a rare type of endometrial cancer that has features of both carcinoma and sarcoma.

Most often, two or more drugs are combined for treatment. Combination chemotherapy works better than one drug alone. The most common combinations include carboplatin/paclitaxel and cisplatin/doxorubicin. Carboplatin/docetaxel and cisplatin/paclitaxel/doxorubicin may be used less often.

Chemotherapy is usually given in cycles: a period of treatment, followed by a rest period. The chemotherapy drugs may be given on one or more days in each cycle. The number of cycles and the length of each cycle depend on the type and dose of drugs, the response to treatment, and the side effects.

The benefits of chemotherapy for endometrial cancer are:

- It can kill any cancer cells that may have spread beyond the uterus, or that may have been left behind after surgery.
- It can lower the risk of recurrence, or delay the recurrence, especially for patients with high-risk or advanced endometrial cancer.

- It can improve the chances of survival, or prolong the survival time, by slowing down the growth and spread of the cancer.
- It can relieve the symptoms of endometrial cancer, such as bleeding, pain, or pressure.

The risks of chemotherapy for endometrial cancer are:

- It can cause side effects, such as hair loss, mouth sores, loss of appetite, vomiting, low blood cell counts, or nerve damage. These side effects depend on the drugs used, the dose, and the duration of treatment. Most of the side effects are temporary and can be managed with medications or supportive care. Some side effects, such as nerve damage or heart damage, may be permanent or long-lasting.
- It can cause complications, such as infections, bleeding, or allergic reactions. These complications can be serious and require immediate medical attention. Some complications, such as kidney damage or

hearing loss, may be permanent or long-lasting.

- It can affect the fertility and the hormone production of the patient, especially for women who have not reached menopause. Chemotherapy can damage the ovaries and cause them to stop producing eggs and hormones, which can lead to infertility or early menopause. This can cause symptoms such as hot flashes, vaginal dryness, mood changes, or osteoporosis. Some women may be able to preserve their fertility by freezing their eggs or embryos before chemotherapy or by using drugs that temporarily stop the ovaries from working during chemotherapy.

These are the main benefits and risks of chemotherapy for endometrial cancer, but they are not the only ones. Each patient may have a different response and experience with chemotherapy, depending on their individual situation and preferences. Therefore, it is important to discuss the benefits and risks of chemotherapy with your doctor and to consider factors such as the effectiveness, the side effects, the cost, and the quality of life.

Hormone Therapy

Hormone therapy is a treatment option for endometrial cancer that uses drugs to block or lower the levels of hormones, such as estrogen and progesterone, that can stimulate the growth of some types of endometrial cancer. It can be given by mouth, by injection, or by implant.

Hormone therapy can be used before surgery to shrink the tumor, especially for young patients who want to preserve their fertility, or after surgery to lower the risk of recurrence, especially for patients with low-risk or early-stage endometrial cancer.

It can also be used for patients who cannot have surgery, radiation therapy, or chemotherapy or for patients whose cancer has spread to distant organs or come back after initial treatment. Hormone therapy may cause some side effects, such as weight gain, fluid retention, hot flashes, vaginal dryness, or mood changes.

Here, we will discuss the different types of hormone therapy drugs for endometrial cancer and their benefits and risks.

Progestins

The primary hormone therapy for endometrial cancer uses progesterone or drugs like it (called progestins). The 2 most commonly used progestins are:

1. Medroxyprogesterone acetate (Provera®), which can be given as an injection or as a pill
2. Megestrol acetate (Megace®), which is given as a pill or liquid

These drugs slow the growth of endometrial cancer cells. They have been found to be useful in treating women with endometrial cancer who want to be able to get pregnant in the future, and this is an area of research interest.

The benefits of progestin therapy for endometrial cancer are:

- It can shrink the tumor or make it disappear, especially for patients with early-stage and low-grade endometrial cancer.
- It can preserve the fertility and the menstrual function of the patient, allowing her to have children in the future.

- It can lower the risk of recurrence or delay the recurrence, especially for patients with low-risk or early-stage endometrial cancer.

The risks of progestin therapy for endometrial cancer are:

- It can cause side effects, such as weight gain, fluid retention, hot flashes, vaginal dryness, or mood changes.
- It can increase the risk of blood clots, especially for patients with other risk factors, such as obesity, smoking, or a history of blood clots.
- It can increase the risk of breast cancer, especially for patients who use progestin for a long time or at high doses.

Tamoxifen

Tamoxifen is an anti-estrogen drug often used to treat breast cancer. It might also be used to treat advanced or recurrent endometrial cancer. Alternating progesterone and tamoxifen is an option that seems to work well and be better tolerated than progesterone alone.

The goal of tamoxifen therapy is to keep any estrogens in the woman's body from boosting the growth of the cancer cells. Though tamoxifen may keep estrogen from *"feeding"* the cancer cells, it acts like a weak estrogen in other body parts. It doesn't cause bone loss, but it can cause hot flashes and vaginal dryness. Women taking tamoxifen also are at higher risk for serious blood clots in the legs.

The benefits of tamoxifen therapy for endometrial cancer are:

- It can slow down the growth or shrink the tumor, especially for patients with advanced or recurrent endometrial cancer.
- It can improve the effectiveness or reduce the side effects of progestin therapy when used in combination or alternation.
- It can prevent bone loss, which can occur with other hormone therapies or menopause.

The risks of tamoxifen therapy for endometrial cancer are:

- It can cause side effects, such as hot flashes, vaginal dryness, or nausea.

- It can increase the risk of blood clots, especially for patients with other risk factors, such as obesity, smoking, or a history of blood clots.
- It can increase the risk of endometrial cancer, especially for patients who use tamoxifen for a long time or at high doses.

Luteinizing hormone-releasing hormone agonists

Luteinizing hormone-releasing hormone agonists (LHRH agonists) are drugs that lower estrogen levels in women who still have working ovaries. They do this by blocking the brain signals telling the ovaries to make estrogen. LHRH agonists are given by injection or implant under the skin. They are often used for carcinosarcoma, a rare type of endometrial cancer that has features of both carcinoma and sarcoma.

The benefits of LHRH agonist therapy for endometrial cancer are:

- It can lower the levels of estrogen, which can stimulate the growth of some types of endometrial cancer.

- It can improve the chances of cure or prevent the cancer from coming back, especially when combined with surgery or chemotherapy.
- It can shrink the tumor or make it disappear, especially for patients with carcinosarcoma.

The risks of LHRH agonist therapy for endometrial cancer are:

- It can cause side effects, such as hot flashes, vaginal dryness, mood changes, or osteoporosis.
- It can cause temporary or permanent infertility, as the ovaries stop producing eggs and hormones.
- It can increase the risk of heart disease, diabetes, or high blood pressure due to low estrogen levels.

Aromatase inhibitors

Aromatase inhibitors (AIs) are drugs that lower estrogen levels in women who have gone through menopause. They do this by blocking the enzyme aromatase, which converts other hormones into estrogen. AIs are given by mouth. They are often used for endometrial cancer that has a certain genetic mutation or biomarker, such as mismatch repair deficiency (dMMR), microsatellite instability-high (MSI-H), or programmed death-ligand 1 (PD-L1).

The benefits of AI therapy for endometrial cancer are:

- It can lower the levels of estrogen that can stimulate the growth of some types of endometrial cancer.
- It can slow down the growth or shrink the tumor, especially for patients with advanced or recurrent endometrial cancer that has a certain genetic mutation or biomarker.
- It can cause fewer or different side effects than other hormone therapies, such as progestins or tamoxifen.

The risks of AI therapy for endometrial cancer are:

- It can cause side effects, such as hot flashes, vaginal dryness, joint pain, or osteoporosis.
- It can increase the risk of heart disease, diabetes, or high cholesterol, due to the low estrogen levels.

- It can interact with other drugs, such as anticoagulants, antidepressants, or supplements, and affect their effectiveness or safety.

These are the main types of hormone therapy for endometrial cancer, but they are not the only ones. Other types of hormone therapy may include progestin-releasing intrauterine devices (IUDs), which can be used for endometrial hyperplasia or early endometrial cancers, or selective estrogen receptor modulators (SERMs), which can block the effects of estrogen on some tissues and mimic them on others.

Targeted Therapy

Targeted therapy is a treatment option for endometrial cancer that uses drugs to target specific changes or features of the cancer cells, such as genes, proteins, or blood vessels.

Targeted therapy drugs work differently from standard chemotherapy drugs, and they tend to have different and sometimes less severe side effects. Targeted therapy is still fairly new in the treatment of endometrial cancer, and only a few drugs are currently approved or available. However, many more drugs are being studied in clinical trials.

Here, we will discuss the different types of targeted therapy drugs for endometrial cancer and their benefits and risks.

Angiogenesis inhibitors

Angiogenesis inhibitors block the formation of new blood vessels that feed the tumor. By cutting off the blood supply, these drugs can slow down or stop the growth and spread of the cancer. Some of the angiogenesis inhibitors that can be used to treat endometrial cancer are:

- **Lenvatinib (Lenvima):** This drug is a type of kinase inhibitor, which means it blocks certain enzymes called kinases that are involved in cell growth, division, and survival. Lenvatinib can also target some proteins that signal new blood vessels to form, such as VEGF and FGF. Lenvatinib is approved to be used along with the immunotherapy drug pembrolizumab (Keytruda) for advanced or recurrent endometrial cancer that is not

MSI-H or dMMR and that has been treated with at least one other type of therapy1. Lenvatinib is taken in capsules once a day. Common side effects include high blood pressure, fatigue, diarrhea, decreased appetite, weight loss, nausea, vomiting, and mouth sores. Less common but more serious side effects can include severe bleeding, blood clots, liver damage, kidney damage, heart failure, and holes in the intestines.

- **Bevacizumab (Avastin):** This drug is a type of monoclonal antibody, which means it is an artificial version of an immune system protein that can bind to a specific target on the cancer cells or the surrounding tissues. Bevacizumab binds to VEGF, a protein that signals new blood vessels to form and prevents it from activating its receptor. Bevacizumab is often given along with chemotherapy, but it can also be given alone for advanced or recurrent endometrial cancer that has been treated with at least one other type of therapy2. Bevacizumab is given as an infusion into a vein (IV) every 2 to 3 weeks. Common side effects include high blood pressure, tiredness, bleeding, low white blood cell counts, headaches, mouth sores, loss of appetite, and diarrhea. Rare but possibly serious side effects include blood clots, severe bleeding, slow wound healing, holes in the colon, and the formation of abnormal connections between the bowel and the skin or bladder.

mTOR inhibitors

mTOR inhibitors are drugs that block a protein called mTOR, which normally helps cells grow and divide. By blocking mTOR, these drugs can stop or slow down the growth of endometrial cancer cells. Some of the mTOR inhibitors that can be used to treat endometrial cancer are:

- **Everolimus (Afinitor):** This drug is approved to be used along with the hormone therapy drug letrozole (Femara) for advanced or recurrent endometrial cancer that is hormone receptor-positive and HER2-negative and that has been treated with hormone therapy before. Everolimus is taken as a tablet once a day. Common side effects include mouth sores, infections, rash, fatigue, diarrhea, and loss of appetite. Less common but more serious side effects can include lung problems, kidney problems, liver problems, high blood sugar, and low blood cell counts.

- **Temsirolimus (Torisel):** This drug is often used for carcinosarcoma, a rare type of endometrial cancer that has features of both carcinoma and sarcoma. It can be given alone or along with chemotherapy for advanced or recurrent carcinosarcoma that has been treated with surgery or radiation before. Temsirolimus is given as an infusion into a vein (IV) once a week. Common side effects include rash, mouth sores, nausea, weakness, swelling, and high blood sugar. Less common but more serious side effects can include lung problems, kidney problems, liver problems, infections, and low blood cell counts.

Aromatase inhibitors

Aromatase inhibitors are drugs that lower the levels of estrogen in women who have gone through menopause. They do this by blocking an enzyme called aromatase, which converts other hormones into estrogen. Lowering estrogen levels can slow down or stop the growth of endometrial cancer cells that depend on estrogen for growth. Some of the aromatase inhibitors that can be used to treat endometrial cancer are:

- **Letrozole (Femara):** This drug is approved to be used along with the mTOR inhibitor everolimus (Afinitor) for advanced or recurrent endometrial cancer that is hormone receptor-positive and HER2-negative, and that has been treated with hormone therapy before3. Letrozole is taken as a tablet once a day. Common side effects include hot flashes, joint pain, fatigue, and nausea. Less common but more serious side effects can include bone loss, high cholesterol, and heart problems.
- **Anastrozole (Arimidex):** This drug is often used for endometrial cancer with a certain genetic mutation or biomarker, such as dMMR, MSI-H, or PD-L1. It can be given alone or along with other targeted therapy or immunotherapy drugs for advanced or recurrent endometrial cancer that has been

treated with other types of therapy before. Anastrozole is taken as a tablet once a day. Common side effects include hot flashes, joint pain, fatigue, and nausea. Less common but more serious side effects can include bone loss, high cholesterol, and heart problems.

These are the main types of targeted therapy drugs for endometrial cancer, but they are not the only ones. Other types of targeted therapy drugs may include kinase inhibitors, monoclonal antibodies, or PARP inhibitors. The best type of targeted therapy for each patient depends on their situation and preferences.

Immunotherapy

Immunotherapy is a treatment option for endometrial cancer that uses drugs to help the body's immune system recognize and kill cancer cells. Immunotherapy can be used for advanced or recurrent endometrial cancer that has been treated with other types of therapy before or for endometrial cancer that has certain genetic changes or biomarkers that make it more likely to respond to immunotherapy.

Immunotherapy may cause side effects, such as fatigue, rash, fever, or diarrhea. Here, we will discuss the different types of immunotherapy drugs for endometrial cancer and their benefits and risks.

Immune checkpoint inhibitors

Immune checkpoint inhibitors are drugs that target proteins in immune cells or cancer cells that usually act as brakes or switches to regulate the immune response. By blocking these proteins, these drugs can boost the immune response against cancer cells. Some of the immune checkpoint inhibitors that can be used to treat endometrial cancer are:

- **Pembrolizumab (Keytruda):** This drug targets PD-1, a protein on immune cells called T cells that normally helps keep them from attacking other cells in the body. By blocking PD-1, pembrolizumab can help T cells recognize and kill cancer cells. Pembrolizumab can be used by itself or along with the targeted drug lenvatinib (Lenvima) for advanced or recurrent endometrial cancer that has been treated with at least one other type of therapy before. Pembrolizumab can also be used for endometrial cancer that has a high level of microsatellite instability (MSI-H), a defect in a mismatch repair gene (dMMR), a high tumor mutational burden (TMB-H), or a high expression of PD-L1, which are biomarkers that indicate a higher likelihood of response to immunotherapy. Pembrolizumab is given as an intravenous (IV) infusion, typically once every 3 or 6 weeks. Common side effects include fatigue, rash, itching, nausea, diarrhea, and cough. Less common but more serious side effects can include severe inflammation of the lungs, liver, kidneys, intestines, skin, or other organs, which can be life-threatening.

- **Dostarlimab (Jemperli):** This drug also targets PD-1 and works in a similar way as pembrolizumab. Dostarlimab can be used by itself or along with chemotherapy for advanced or recurrent endometrial cancer that has been treated with at least one other type of therapy before. Dostarlimab can also be used for endometrial cancer that has a defect in a mismatch repair gene (dMMR) or a high level of microsatellite instability

(MSI-H), which are biomarkers that indicate a higher likelihood of response to immunotherapy. Dostarlimab is given as an intravenous (IV) infusion, typically once every 3 weeks at first and then every 6 weeks. Common side effects include fatigue, nausea, diarrhea, rash, and itching. Less common but more serious side effects can include severe inflammation of the lungs, liver, kidneys, intestines, skin, or other organs, which can be life-threatening.

The benefits of immunotherapy for endometrial cancer are:

- It can shrink the tumor or make it disappear, especially for patients with endometrial cancer that have certain genetic changes or biomarkers that make it more likely to respond to immunotherapy.
- It can lower the risk of recurrence or delay the recurrence, especially for patients with advanced or recurrent endometrial cancer that has been treated with other types of therapy before.

- It can improve the chances of survival or prolong the survival time by slowing down the growth and spread of the cancer.
- It can cause fewer or different side effects than other types of therapy, such as chemotherapy or hormone therapy.

The risks of immunotherapy for endometrial cancer are:

- It can cause side effects, such as fatigue, rash, fever, or diarrhea, affecting the patient's quality of life.
- It can cause complications, such as severe inflammation of the lungs, liver, kidneys, intestines, skin, or other organs, which can be life-threatening and require immediate medical attention.
- It can interact with other drugs, such as steroids, antibiotics, or vaccines, and affect their effectiveness or safety.
- It can be expensive, and not all insurance plans may cover the cost of immunotherapy.

Clinical Trials

Clinical trials are research studies that test new treatments or procedures for endometrial cancer. Clinical trials can offer patients access to cutting-edge therapies not widely available elsewhere and contribute to advancing medical knowledge and practice. However, clinical trials also have risks and limitations, such as possible side effects, unknown outcomes, eligibility criteria, and extra costs or time commitments.

Here, we will discuss the different types of clinical trials for endometrial cancer and their benefits and risks.

Types of Clinical Trials

There are different types of clinical trials for endometrial cancer depending on their purpose and phase, such as prevention, diagnosis, and treatment.

- **Treatment trials:** These trials test new drugs, combinations of drugs, or new ways of giving drugs, such as oral, intravenous, or intraperitoneal. They also test new types of therapy, such as surgery, radiation, hormone therapy, targeted therapy, immunotherapy, or gene therapy. Treatment trials aim to find out if a new treatment is safe and effective and how it compares to the standard treatment.

- **Prevention trials:** These trials test new ways of preventing endometrial cancer, such as vaccines, drugs, dietary supplements, or lifestyle changes. Prevention trials aim to find out if a new intervention can lower the risk of developing endometrial cancer or delay its onset in people who have not had the disease before.

- **Screening trials:** These trials test new ways of detecting endometrial cancer, such as blood tests, imaging tests, or genetic tests. Screening trials aim to find out if a new test can find endometrial cancer early when it is more likely to be cured or prevent it from progressing to a more advanced stage.

- **Diagnostic trials:** These trials test new ways of diagnosing endometrial cancer, such as biomarkers, molecular tests, or tissue samples. Diagnostic trials aim to find out if a new test can accurately identify the type, stage, grade, or subtype of endometrial cancer or predict its response to treatment or prognosis.

- **Supportive care trials:** These trials test new ways of improving the quality of life of endometrial cancer patients, such as pain management, symptom control, psychological support, or palliative care. Supportive care trials aim to find out if a new intervention can reduce the physical, emotional, or social burden of endometrial cancer or enhance the well-being of patients and their caregivers.

Clinical trials are also classified by their phase, which indicates the stage of development and the study's goal. The phases of clinical trials are:

- **Phase 0:** These are very small studies that test a new drug or procedure in a few people, usually less than 15, for the first time. They aim to find out how the drug or procedure works in the body and what dose is safe and effective. Phase 0 trials are rare, and they do not measure the effectiveness of the drug or procedure.

- **Phase I:** These are small studies that test a new drug or procedure in a small group of people, usually 15 to 30, who have endometrial cancer or other types of cancer. They aim to find out the best way to give the drug or procedure, the highest dose that can be given safely, and the possible side effects. Phase I trials are not designed to measure the effectiveness of the drug or procedure. However, some may show early signs of benefit.

- **Phase II:** These are larger studies that test a new drug or procedure in a larger group of people, usually 100 to 300, who have endometrial cancer or a specific subtype of endometrial cancer. They aim to find out if the drug or procedure works for endometrial cancer and the optimal dose and schedule. Phase II trials also monitor the drug's or procedure's safety and side effects. Some phase II trials may compare the new drug or procedure to the standard or a placebo (a dummy treatment).

- **Phase III:** These are large studies that test a new drug or procedure in a very large group of people, usually several hundred to thousands, who have endometrial cancer or a specific subtype of endometrial cancer. They aim to compare the new drug or procedure to the standard treatment or a placebo and find out which is better regarding safety and effectiveness. Phase III trials also measure the impact of the new drug or procedure on the quality of life, survival, and recurrence of endometrial cancer. Phase III trials are usually randomized, meaning the participants are assigned to the new drug or procedure, or the standard treatment or placebo, by chance. They are also usually double-blind, meaning the participants and the researchers know who gets which treatment at the end of the study. Phase III trials are the most rigorous and conclusive type of clinical trials, and they are required before a new drug or procedure can be approved for general use.

- **Phase IV:** These studies test a new drug or procedure after it has been approved for general use and is available on the market. They aim to monitor the long-term safety and effectiveness of the drug or procedure and to discover any new side effects, interactions, or benefits. Phase IV trials may also compare the new drug or procedure to other treatments or explore new ways of using it, such as different doses, schedules, or combinations.

The benefits of clinical trials for endometrial cancer are:

- They can offer patients access to new and innovative treatments or procedures that are not widely available elsewhere and that may be more effective or less toxic than the standard treatment.
- They can provide patients with high-quality care and close monitoring by a team of experts who follow strict protocols and guidelines to ensure the safety and well-being of the participants.
- They can contribute to advancing medical knowledge and practice and help improve the outcomes and quality of life of future endometrial cancer patients.

The risks of clinical trials for endometrial cancer are:

- They can cause side effects or complications, which may be unknown, unexpected, or worse than the standard treatment. Some side effects or complications may be severe or life-threatening and require additional treatment or hospitalization.

- They may only work for some patients or not as well as the standard treatment. Some patients may not benefit from the new treatment or procedure or may experience disease progression or recurrence.

- They may have eligibility criteria, which are patients' requirements to join the study. These criteria may include age, gender, type, stage, grade, or subtype of endometrial cancer, previous treatments, medical history, or other factors. Some patients may not qualify for the study or may be excluded for various reasons.

- They may have extra costs or time commitments, which may not be covered by insurance or reimbursed by the study sponsor. These costs or commitments may include travel expenses, co-payments, tests, procedures, or visits not part of the standard care. Some patients may have to stop working or change their daily routine to participate in the study.

Clinical trials for endometrial cancer have varying benefits and risks depending on the purpose, phase, and study design. Discussing these factors with your doctor and considering eligibility, treatment, outcome, cost, and quality of life is crucial.

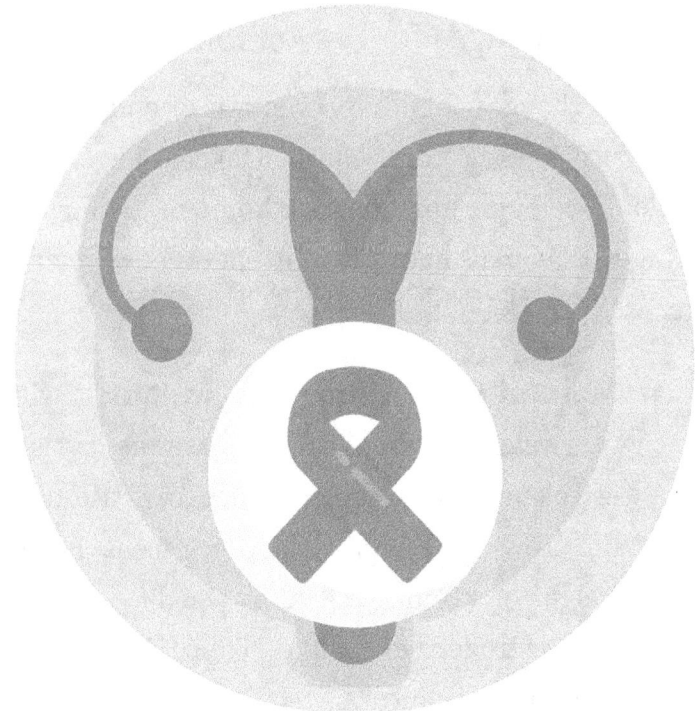

Chapter 6

Prevention Strategies

Lifestyle Changes for Prevention

Lifestyle changes for the prevention of endometrial cancer are actions that you can take to lower your risk of developing this disease. Some of the lifestyle changes that may help prevent endometrial cancer are:

- **Maintaining a healthy weight:** Being overweight or obese can increase the levels of estrogen in your body, which can stimulate the growth of endometrial cancer cells. Losing weight or keeping a healthy weight can lower your estrogen levels and reduce your risk of endometrial cancer.

- **Being physically active:** Physical activity can help you burn calories, lose weight, and lower your estrogen levels. It can also improve your overall health and well-being. Aim for at least 150 minutes of moderate-intensity or 75 minutes of vigorous-intensity physical activity per week, or a combination of both.

- **Limiting the use of hormone therapy:** Hormone therapy, such as estrogen or progestin, can be used to treat the symptoms of menopause, such as hot flashes, vaginal dryness, or osteoporosis. However, hormone therapy can also increase the risk of endometrial cancer, especially if you use estrogen alone or for a long time. If you need hormone therapy, talk to your doctor about the benefits and risks, and use the lowest dose and shortest duration possible. You may also consider using other forms of hormone therapy, such as vaginal creams, rings, or tablets, which deliver lower doses of hormones and may have less effect on the endometrium.

- **Using birth control pills:** Birth control pills, which contain estrogen and progestin, can lower the risk of endometrial cancer by preventing ovulation and reducing the exposure of the endometrium to estrogen. The protective effect of birth control pills lasts for several years after you stop using them. However, birth control pills can also have some side effects and risks, such as blood clots, stroke, or breast cancer. Talk to your doctor about the best birth control option for you.

- **Getting treated for endometrial problems:** Some conditions that affect the endometrium, such as endometrial hyperplasia or polyps, can increase the risk of endometrial cancer. Getting proper treatment for these conditions, such as hormones, surgery, or other procedures, can prevent them from progressing to cancer. If you have abnormal vaginal bleeding, such as bleeding after menopause or between periods, see your doctor and get it checked right away.

Regular Screenings and Early Detection

Regular screenings and early detection of endometrial cancer are important for improving the chances of survival and recovery. However, there is no standard or routine screening test for endometrial cancer, and most cases are found at an early stage because of symptoms such as abnormal vaginal bleeding. Some tests that may help detect endometrial cancer are being studied, such as:

- **Pap test:** This is a test that collects cells from the cervix and checks them for abnormal changes. A Pap test can sometimes find endometrial cancer cells that have spread to the cervix, but it is not a reliable way to screen for endometrial cancer.

- **Transvaginal ultrasound:** This is a test that uses sound waves to create images of the uterus and other pelvic organs. A transvaginal ultrasound can measure the thickness of the endometrium and look for any abnormal growths. A thickened endometrium or a mass may suggest endometrial cancer, but it can also be caused by other conditions, such as polyps or fibroids.

- **Endometrial sampling:** This is a procedure that removes a small piece of tissue from the endometrium and examines it under a microscope. An endometrial sample can confirm the diagnosis of endometrial cancer or rule out other causes of abnormal bleeding. There are different ways to do an endometrial sampling, such as endometrial biopsy, dilation and curettage (D&C), or hysteroscopy.

Screening tests for endometrial cancer are not recommended for all women, but they may be considered for women who have a high risk of developing the disease, such as those who have:

- A family history of endometrial cancer, especially if they have a genetic syndrome that increases the risk, such as Lynch syndrome or Cowden syndrome.
- A personal history of endometrial hyperplasia, which is a condition that causes

the endometrium to grow too thick and become abnormal.

- A history of taking estrogen without progestin for hormone therapy, which can stimulate the growth of the endometrium.

If you have any of these risk factors or if you have any symptoms of endometrial cancer, such as abnormal vaginal bleeding, talk to your doctor about whether you need screening tests for endometrial cancer and how often you should have them. Your doctor will also advise you on how to lower your risk of endometrial cancer.

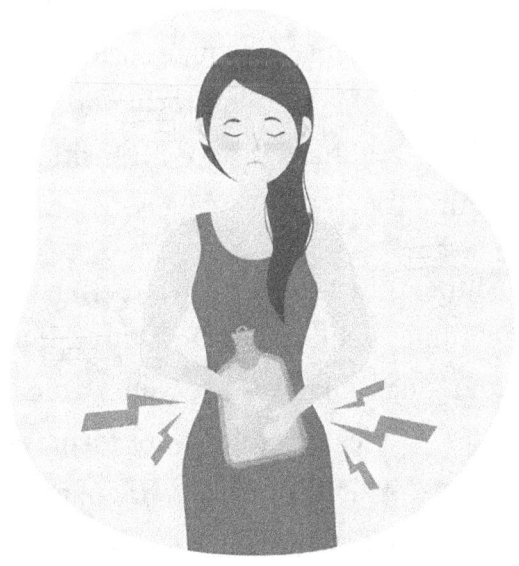

Chapter 7

Navigating Recovery

Post-Treatment Care

Finishing active endometrial cancer treatment ushers in the recovery phase, but the journey does not end there. Post-treatment care focuses on managing side effects, monitoring for recurrence, maintaining wellness, and transitioning into survivorship.

Your healthcare team will provide a post-treatment plan detailing required follow-up appointments, tests, and surveillance to watch for potential recurrence. Typically, follow-up visits are more frequent in the first 1-2 years, then may taper to annually or based on patient symptoms.

Physical and emotional changes are expected after cancer treatment. Discuss any persistent or concerning side effects at follow-up visits, like fatigue, urinary issues, lymphodema, pain, depression, anxiety, and sexual changes. Your team can help manage these effects through medication, physical therapy, counseling, and other solutions to improve your quality of life.

Some women may need dilation and curettage, radiation, or hormone treatments if the cancer is estrogen-receptor positive. For advanced-stage cancers, your oncologist may recommend chemotherapy, radiation, or additional surgery after the initial treatment.

Maintaining a healthy lifestyle and diet can promote recovery. Eat nutritious whole foods, exercise as much as possible, manage stress, avoid smoking, and achieve or maintain a healthy weight. Physical activity, even regular short walks, helps build energy and strength.

Listen to your body, and do not overexert. Rest when needed, and build up activity gradually. Get adequate sleep. Join a support group to connect with fellow survivors. Express your emotions; journaling can help. Follow care instructions closely and keep all appointments.

Let your care team know immediately about symptoms like bleeding, weight loss, or persistent pain so any potential recurrence can be assessed promptly. Local recurrences or distant metastases need quick action. Surveillance testing will be scheduled routinely to monitor your condition.

Recovery takes time, but the future remains hopeful. With dedicated self-care, following recommendations, embracing a positive mindset, and attending all follow-ups, you can move successfully into cancer survivorship.

Physical and Emotional Recovery

Coping with the physical and emotional changes that accompany endometrial cancer treatment is an important part of the recovery process. Understanding common challenges and remedies can smooth the transition.

Physically, fatigue is one of survivors' most persistent side effects. Treatment strains the body, so significant exhaustion often lingers even after finishing. Gradually resuming exercise like walking helps counter fatigue, as does maintaining good nutrition. Getting adequate restorative sleep and napping can also alleviate tiredness.

Pain may continue, especially if radiation is part of the treatment protocol. Ask about pain medication options and non-drug therapies like acupuncture, massage, or physical therapy to find relief. Gentle stretching can also ease muscle tightness. Apply ice or heat to painful areas.

Urinary or bowel habit changes are also common after treatment involving radiation. Stay hydrated, and discuss any persistent or worrisome bladder or bowel issues with your care team for solutions. Some dietary modifications, fiber supplements, or medications may help regulate functions. Pelvic floor therapy can also benefit certain urinary problems.

Pay attention to nutrition needs during recovery, as treatment effects and hormonal shifts can affect appetite and eating habits. Work with a nutritionist to develop a healthy meal plan if you are dealing with weight changes. Some find smaller, frequent meals easier to tolerate than three large meals daily.

Emotionally, anxiety and depression frequently occur in the post-treatment adjustment period. You may fear the cancer returning or struggle with body image changes after surgery. Joining a support group to connect with fellow survivors provides reassurance. Consider counseling for mood disorders or lingering trauma. Antidepressants may also help in some cases.

Communicate openly with loved ones about what you are feeling and experiencing. Intimacy and sexual challenges can strain relationships, so have ongoing discussions with your partner. Various medical interventions can help with sexual function if needed.

Expect ups and downs during the recovery and adjustment process. Each person's experience is unique. Give yourself ample time, utilize available resources for support, and know there is hope ahead. With dedication to your physical and emotional well-being, you can thrive after endometrial cancer.

Support Systems and Resources

Support systems and resources are essential for women recovering from endometrial cancer and its treatment. Support systems and resources can provide emotional, practical, and informational assistance and a sense of belonging and empowerment. Support systems and resources can include:

- **Family and friends:** Family and friends are often the primary sources of support for women who have had endometrial cancer and its treatment. They can offer you love, comfort, encouragement, and help with your daily needs, such as transportation, household chores, or childcare. However, family and friends may also have emotions, concerns, or expectations that may affect your relationship with them. You should communicate openly and honestly with your family and friends about your feelings, needs, and boundaries. You should also appreciate their efforts and acknowledge their limitations. You should seek professional help if you have conflicts or difficulties with your family or friends that interfere with your recovery.

- **Healthcare team:** Your healthcare team comprises doctors, nurses, and other professionals involved in your diagnosis, treatment, and follow-up care for endometrial cancer. They can provide medical information, guidance, support, and referrals to other specialists or services you may need. You should maintain a good relationship with your healthcare team by asking questions, expressing your concerns, and following their recommendations. You should also update them on your health status, symptoms, and side effects. You should contact your healthcare team if you have any problems or changes in your condition that require their attention.

- **Support groups:** Support groups are gatherings of people who share similar experiences or challenges related to endometrial cancer or its treatment. They can offer emotional support, practical advice, coping strategies, and a sense of community and solidarity. Professionals, such as social workers or counselors, or peers, such as survivors or caregivers, can lead support groups. Support groups can be held in person, online, or over the phone. You can find support groups through your healthcare team, local hospital, community center, or online platforms, such as the Endometrial Cancer Foundation or SHARE Cancer Support.

- **Counseling and therapy:** Counseling and therapy are professional services that can help you cope with the emotional and psychological aspects of endometrial cancer and its treatment. They can help you deal with stress, anxiety, depression, fear, anger, guilt, grief, or other emotions that may affect your recovery. They can also help you improve your self-esteem, confidence, and resilience, as well as your relationships, sexuality, and fertility. Counseling and therapy can be provided by psychologists, psychiatrists, social workers, or counselors. They can be delivered individually, as a couple, as a family, or as a group. You can find counseling and therapy through your healthcare team, insurance company, employer, or online platforms, such as **Memorial Sloan Kettering Counseling Center** or **Cancer Care.**

- **Education and information:** Education and information are vital for women recovering from endometrial cancer and its treatment. They can help you understand your diagnosis, treatment, and follow-up care, as well as the possible complications and long-term effects of endometrial cancer and its treatment. They can also help you make informed decisions, manage expectations, and plan for the future. Your healthcare team, local library, community center, or online platforms, such as the **American Cancer Society** or **National Cancer Institute,** can provide education and information.

- **Advocacy and research:** Advocacy and research are important for women recovering from endometrial cancer and its treatment. They can help you raise awareness, influence policy, and improve outcomes for endometrial cancer and its treatment. They can also help you contribute to the advancement of knowledge, prevention, and cure for endometrial cancer and its treatment. Advocacy and research can be done by joining or supporting organizations, campaigns, or studies on endometrial cancer and its treatment, such as the **Endometrial Cancer Action Network for African Americans** or **Gynecologic Oncology Group.**

Support systems and resources can include family, friends, the healthcare team, support groups, counseling and therapy, education and information, and advocacy and research. You should seek and use the support systems and resources that suit your needs, preferences, and goals. You should also be open to new or different sources of support and resources that may benefit your recovery. Remember that you are not alone in this journey, and there are many people and organizations that can help you recover and thrive.

Chapter 8

Living with Endometrial Cancer

Managing Side Effects and Symptoms

Living with endometrial cancer often involves dealing with treatment side effects and ongoing symptoms. Working closely with your healthcare providers to manage effects through various interventions can help maintain your quality of life.

- **Fatigue:** This extremely common side effect may persist long after treatment ends. Regular low-to-moderate-intensity exercise, yoga, good sleep habits, nutrition, and stress management help counter fatigue. Rule out other causes, like anemia or thyroid dysfunction.

- **Pain:** If pain like backaches or joint pain lingers, over-the-counter or prescription medications provide relief. Physical therapy, massage, acupuncture, hot/cold therapy, and mindfulness exercises can minimize discomfort.

- **Bowel and Bladder Changes:** If needed, diet adjustments, fiber supplements, probiotics, pelvic floor therapy, timed-voiding schedules, protective pads, and antibiotics assist with treatment-related urinary and bowel issues. Track and communicate symptoms.

- **Sexual Challenges:** Vaginal dryness, erectile dysfunction, lowered desire, discomfort, or difficulty reaching orgasm often occur. Use lubricants, communicate needs, try positioning aids, massage, sensual activities, and therapies like localized estrogen or nerve-sparing surgery.

- **Emotional Distress:** Anxiety, depression, stress, and fear commonly burden cancer patients. Support groups, counseling, psychotherapy, meditation, journaling, and medication, if warranted, can help overcome emotional obstacles.

- **Cognition Changes:** Radiation may impair memory, concentration, multitasking, and processing speed. Compensatory techniques, cognitive rehabilitation, puzzle games, and providing written directions assist with the "chemo brain."

- **Nutrition Issues:** Work with a dietitian to optimize nutrition and weight. Address symptoms like taste changes, nausea, bowel issues, and fatigue through dietary strategies. Hydration is also key.

Ongoing communication with your care team is vital to tailoring symptom management approaches over treatment, recovery, survivorship, and beyond. New therapies continually emerge, so speak up about persistent or concerning effects.

Coping with the Emotional Impact

Significant emotional impacts often accompany the physical toll of endometrial cancer. Anxiety, depression, anger, grief, fear, and trauma are common responses. Building coping strategies helps manage the emotional fallout.

Seeking out mental health support is key. Meet with a counselor or therapist regularly to process emotions in a judgment-free space. Cognitive behavioral therapy and mindfulness-based approaches can lessen anxiety and depressive thinking patterns.

It's crucial to confide in trusted friends and family who listen without trying to diminish your feelings. Be careful in choosing whom to support, as not everyone is emotionally equipped for the role.

Join a support group, either locally or online, to share with others going through similar struggles. Groups focused on art therapy, yoga, or other activities also unite survivors. Knowing you are not alone is comforting.

Consider antidepressant medication if recommended by your doctor. Certain drugs help treat depression, anxiety, sleep disruption, and nerve pain often associated with cancer.

Foster open communication with your treatment team. Be honest about your emotional struggles so they can connect you with resources. Some cancer centers have psychologists on staff.

Make time for self-care through relaxing activities like reading, spending time outdoors, listening to music, enjoying a warm bath, or treating yourself to a massage. Do things solely for you.

Maintain perspective through positive self-talk, affirmations, looking at uplifting images, reading inspirational quotes, or starting a gratitude journal. Counter harmful thought patterns.

Express yourself creatively through art, writing, music, or other outlets. Creating helps you constructively tap into and release emotions.

Learn relaxation techniques like deep breathing, visualization, meditation, and progressive muscle relaxation to calm anxiety. Apps offer guided meditations.

Strengthening emotional resilience takes work, but utilizing available resources makes the process more manageable. With time and coping skills, hope can prevail.

Staying Active and Healthy

Staying active and healthy is a key part of living with endometrial cancer. Being physically active and eating a healthy diet can help you improve your recovery, reduce your risk of recurrence or new cancers, and enhance your quality of life and well-being. Some of the benefits of staying active and healthy are:

- Improving your physical fitness, strength, and flexibility;
- Boosting your immune system and lowering inflammation;
- Balancing your hormones and reducing menopausal symptoms;
- Managing your weight and preventing obesity-related diseases;
- Relieving stress, anxiety, and depression;
- Increasing your energy, mood, and confidence.

Some of the strategies that can help you stay active and healthy are:

- Follow the physical activity guidelines for cancer survivors. The American Cancer Society recommends that cancer survivors should:
  - Build up to 150–300 minutes of moderate (or 75–150 minutes of vigorous-intensity) activity each week. Exercise several times a week for at least 10 minutes at a time. Include resistance training exercises at least 2 days per week. Do stretching exercises at least 2 days each week.
  - Choose activities that you enjoy, and that suit your abilities and preferences. You can try walking, jogging, cycling, swimming, dancing, or gardening. You can also join a fitness class, a sports team, or a walking group.
  - Start slowly and gradually increase the intensity and duration of your exercise. Listen to your body and adjust your pace and frequency according to your

energy level, symptoms, and side effects. Rest when you need to and avoid overexertion.

o Talk to your doctor before starting or changing your exercise routine. Your doctor can help you set realistic and safe goals and advise you on any precautions or limitations that you may have. You may also benefit from working with a physical therapist, an exercise physiologist, or a personal trainer with cancer patient experience.

- Follow a healthy eating pattern that includes plenty of fruits, vegetables, and whole grains, and limit or avoid red and processed meats, sugary drinks, and highly processed foods. The American Cancer Society recommends that cancer survivors should:

  o Eat at least 2 ½ cups of vegetables and fruits daily. Choose various colors and types to get a range of nutrients and antioxidants. Include dark green, leafy, and cruciferous vegetables, such as broccoli, kale, cabbage, and cauliflower. Limit your intake of starchy vegetables, such as potatoes, corn, and peas.

○ Choose whole grains over refined grains. Whole grains contain more fiber, vitamins, minerals, and phytochemicals than refined grains. Aim for at least 3 servings of whole grains daily, such as whole wheat bread, brown rice, oats, quinoa, or barley.

○ Limit your intake of red meat and processed meat. Red meat includes beef, pork, lamb, and goat. Processed meat includes bacon, ham, sausage, hot dogs, and deli meats. These meats can increase your risk of colorectal cancer and other chronic diseases. Aim for no more than 18 ounces of cooked red meat per week, and avoid or limit processed meat as much as possible.

○ Avoid or limit sugary drinks and foods. Sugary drinks and foods include soft drinks, fruit juices, sports drinks, energy drinks, cakes, cookies, candy, and ice cream. These foods can add extra calories and sugar to your diet and increase your risk of obesity, diabetes, and heart disease. Choose water, unsweetened tea, or coffee as your main beverages, and limit your intake of added sugars to no more than 10% of your total calories per day.

o Avoid or limit highly processed foods. Highly processed foods include chips, crackers, pretzels, instant noodles, frozen meals, canned soups, and sauces. These foods are often high in salt, fat, sugar, and additives and low in nutrients and fiber. They can increase your risk of high blood pressure, high cholesterol, and heart disease. Choose fresh, whole, or minimally processed foods as much as possible, and read the nutrition labels and ingredient lists carefully.

- Drink enough water to stay hydrated. Water is essential for your body's functions, such as digestion, circulation, temperature regulation, and waste elimination. Water can also help you control your appetite, prevent constipation, and flush out toxins. Aim for at least 8 glasses of water daily, or more if you exercise, sweat, or have diarrhea or vomiting. You can also drink other fluids, such as herbal teas, soups, or milk, but avoid or limit caffeinated, alcoholic, or sugary drinks, as they can dehydrate you or add extra calories to your diet.

- Take dietary supplements only if advised by your doctor. Dietary supplements include vitamins, minerals, herbs, or other substances taken by mouth to supplement your diet. Some dietary supplements help you meet your nutritional needs, especially if you have a poor appetite, food allergies, or dietary restrictions. However, some dietary supplements may also interact with your medications, affect your hormone levels, or increase your risk of bleeding or other complications. Therefore, you should consult your doctor before taking any dietary supplements. Your doctor can help you determine if you need any supplements and what type, dose, and duration are appropriate.

Adjusting to a "new normal" with cancer takes time. Having patience and self-compassion helps. Making self-care and healthy routines high priorities supports living well.

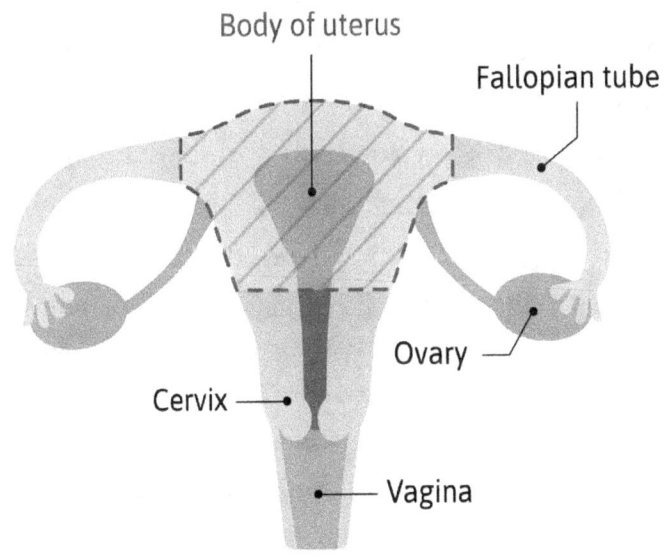

Body of uterus

Fallopian tube

Ovary

Cervix

Vagina

Partial hysterectomy

Conclusion

In this book, you have learned about endometrial cancer, a type of cancer that starts in the lining of the uterus. You now know the causes, risk factors, symptoms, diagnosis, treatment, and recovery of endometrial cancer. You have also learned about the physical and emotional challenges that you may face while living with endometrial cancer and how to cope with them. You have also learned about the support systems and resources available to you and your loved ones.

Endometrial cancer is the most common gynecologic cancer in women, affecting about 1 in 37 women in their lifetime. However, endometrial cancer is also one of the most treatable and curable cancers, especially if detected early. The survival rate for endometrial cancer is high, and many women go on to live long and healthy lives after the treatment.

The Future of Endometrial Cancer Treatment
As research progresses, new therapies that improve outcomes for endometrial cancer patients continue to emerge. In the future, treatment is likely to become ever more personalized and targeted.

Immunotherapies that rally the body's immune system against cancer cells may soon revolutionize treatment, especially for advanced endometrial cancer. Checkpoint inhibitors, therapeutic vaccines, and monoclonal antibodies are among the burgeoning immunotherapies being studied in clinical trials.

Targeted drug therapies that attack specific molecules and genes crucial for tumor growth and survival also hold great promise. These novel agents will provide oncologists with an expanding arsenal.

Advanced surgical techniques, like robotic surgery, are enhancing precision and minimally invasive options for hysterectomies and lymph node removal.

Faster recovery and fewer complications give patients more choices.

Exciting new therapies continue to emerge from dedicated researchers. The future remains bright for more effective endometrial cancer treatment tailored to each woman's specific cancer characteristics.

Final Thoughts and Encouragement

Thank you for joining me in exploring endometrial cancer from various angles. I hope you now feel equipped with a fuller understanding and a trove of resources to draw upon. Although the road ahead has challenges, knowledge, and support light the way. You are stronger than you know.

This disease does not define you. Keep sight of who you are at your core—that inner light shines as brightly as ever. Surround yourself with positive people who will uplift you. And most importantly, never give up hope. Hope is what carries us through dark times into light. You are brave, you are resilient, and you will overcome this. Keep persevering one step at a time, one day at a time. I wish you all the best in your recovery and beyond. You've got this!

Glossary

A glossary can help you understand the meaning and usage of unfamiliar words or concepts. Here is a glossary of some common terms related to endometrial cancer:

- **Adenocarcinoma:** A type of cancer that starts in the cells that line certain organs or tissues, such as the endometrium (the lining of the uterus).
- **Biopsy:** A procedure that involves taking a small tissue sample from the body and examining it under a microscope to check for cancer or other abnormalities.
- **Chemotherapy:** A type of cancer treatment that uses drugs to kill cancer cells or stop them from growing and dividing.

- **Endometrial cancer:** A type of cancer that starts in the endometrium (the lining of the uterus). It is the most common gynecologic cancer in women.

- **Endometrium:** The inner layer of tissue that lines the uterus. It thickens and sheds monthly during the menstrual cycle unless a pregnancy occurs.

- **Estrogen:** A hormone produced mainly by the ovaries in women. It regulates the menstrual cycle and affects the development and function of the female reproductive organs. It also affects other body parts, such as the bones, the heart, and the brain.

- **Hysterectomy:** A surgery that involves removing the uterus. Sometimes, other organs or structures, such as the ovaries, the fallopian tubes, the cervix, or the lymph nodes, may also be removed.

- **Immunotherapy:** A type of cancer treatment that uses substances that stimulate or enhance the immune system's ability to fight cancer cells.

- **Lymph nodes:** Small, bean-shaped structures that are part of the lymphatic system. They filter and store lymph, a clear fluid that carries white blood cells and other substances that help fight infections and diseases. They also trap and destroy cancer cells or other foreign substances that enter the lymphatic system.

- **Menopause:** The time in a woman's life when her ovaries stop producing eggs and hormones, and her menstrual periods stop permanently. Menopause usually occurs around the age of 50, but it can vary depending on various factors, such as genetics, health, or lifestyle.

- **Metastasis:** The spread of cancer from its original site to other parts of the body through the blood or the lymphatic system.

- **Progesterone:** A hormone produced mainly by women's ovaries. It prepares the endometrium for the implantation of a fertilized egg and supports pregnancy. It also affects other body parts, such as the breasts, the skin, and the mood.

- **Radiation therapy:** A type of cancer treatment that uses high-energy rays or particles to damage or destroy cancer cells or stop them from growing and dividing.
- **Recurrence:** The return of cancer after a period of remission or after the completion of treatment.
- **Remission:** The disappearance or reduction of the signs and symptoms of cancer, either partially or completely. Remission can be temporary or permanent, depending on the type and stage of the cancer and the effectiveness of the treatment.
- **Staging:** The process of determining the extent and spread of cancer in the body. Staging helps plan the treatment and predict the prognosis of cancer. Staging is usually based on the tumor's size and location, the lymph nodes' involvement, and the presence or absence of metastasis.
- **Surgery:** A type of cancer treatment that involves removing the tumor and some surrounding normal tissue from the body. Surgery can be used to diagnose, treat, or

prevent cancer or to relieve symptoms or complications caused by cancer.

- **Targeted therapy:** A type of cancer treatment that uses drugs or other substances that target and block specific molecules or pathways involved in cancer cell growth and spread. Targeted therapy can help stop or slow down the cancer and spare the normal cells.

- **Uterus:** A hollow, pear-shaped organ that is part of the female reproductive system. It is where a fetus develops and grows during pregnancy. It is also where the endometrium is located.

References

Here are some of the references that I used to write this book:

1. American Cancer Society. (2020). Endometrial Cancer. Retrieved from https://www.cancer.org/cancer/endometrial-cancer.html

2. National Cancer Institute. (2020). Endometrial Cancer Treatment (PDQ®)–Patient Version. Retrieved from https://www.cancer.gov/types/uterine/patient/endometrial-treatment-pdq

3. Mayo Clinic. (2020). Endometrial cancer. Retrieved from https://www.mayoclinic.org/diseases-conditions/endometrial-cancer/symptoms-causes/syc-20352461

4. Memorial Sloan Kettering Cancer Center. (2020). Living Beyond Uterine (Endometrial) Cancer. Retrieved from https://www.mskcc.org/cancer-care/types/uterine/living-beyond

5. Endometrial Cancer Foundation. (2020). Retrieved from https://www.endometrialcancer.org/

6. SHARE Cancer Support. (2020). Uterine Cancer Support. Retrieved from https://www.sharecancersupport.org/uterine-cancer-support/

7. Cancer Care. (2020). Endometrial Cancer. Retrieved from https://www.cancercare.org/diagnosis/endometrial_cancer

8. Endometrial Cancer Action Network for African Americans. (2020). Retrieved from https://ecanawomen.org/

9. Gynecologic Oncology Group. (2020). Retrieved from https://gog.org/